Dental Implants

A Guide for the General Practitioner

Michael Norton BDS

London, England

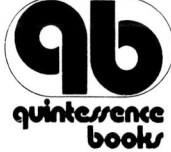

Quintessence Publishing Co Ltd
London, Berlin, Chicago, São Paulo, Tokyo, Moscow,
Prague and Warsaw

First published 1995 by
Quintessence Publishing Company Ltd
London, UK

British Library Cataloguing in Publication Data
Norton, Michael
 Dental Implants
 1. Prosthetic dentistry
 I. Title
 617.69

 ISBN 1-85097-037-8

Printed and bound by Toppan Printing Co Pte Ltd, Singapore
Litho production by Toppan Printing Co Pte Ltd, Singapore

Typesetting by Alacrity Phototypesetters,
Banwell Castle, Weston-super-Mare, UK.

Foreword

It must be recognised that implants have become part of the mainstream of available dental treatment, and the time has passed when a dentist could describe implants to his patients as "experimental". So much well documented evidence now exists of the long term success of osseointegrated fixtures that it could well amount to negligent care if a practitioner fails to mention the possibility of implants to a patient who might benefit from such treatment.

Until now there has been a clear need for a book introducing the general practitioner to the implant field. Michael Norton's book answers this need, giving the general practitioner a most valuable insight into implantology, although it goes without saying that no one should even think of starting in the implant field without intensive study, including attendance at recognised courses of hands-on instruction.

Several books exist which are aimed at the specialist but nothing has been published before that gives the general practitioner such a comprehensive overview of implant dentistry, with guidance as to patient selection and a clear understanding of exactly how patients may benefit from implants. That gap is now filled by this admirably clear and concise and extremely readable book. Mysteries and possible misconceptions are cleared up and the practitioner will find guidance as to exactly how far he actively wants to become involved in this most exciting field.

Although Michael Norton mostly describes procedures with the very simple and logical Astra-Tech system, his wise observations and descriptions apply to most other systems as well.

This is a volume that the conscientious practitioner cannot afford to ignore.

Colin Hall Dexter
Past Chairman, British
Dental Health Foundation

Acknowledgements

There are many dental colleagues, technicians and friends who will have directly or indirectly contributed to the compilation of this text. None of the cases demonstrated could have been completed without the help and skill of colleagues, to whom equal acknowledgement is due.

I would also like to thank all my colleagues and friends within Astra Tech, for their support and encouragement over the years and in particular during the writing of this book.

I am in your debt.

Michael Norton

Dedicated to
my wife Louise, parents and family,
with love and thanks
for all your support and encouragement

Introduction

Why Implants?

Since the publication of the recommendations on the consensus development conference on dental implants in 1979,[1] and the 15 year results published by Adell et al. in 1981,[2] implantology has taken centre stage as a well researched and predictable treatment modality. For those already offering this treatment, the successful rehabilitation of patients with endosseous implants seems to confirm this predictability. Furthermore the attitude of patients and their degree of satisfaction is well documented,[3-6] with clear evidence that it improves their self confidence and quality of life.[7]

The significance of implantology for the profession, runs deeper than simply offering a new therapy. As an alternative, it challenges and augments the conventional treatment plan, presenting greater opportunities to conserve hard and soft tissues. It is this concept that lends such significance to implantology and the role it should now play in general dental practice.

The GDP, The Specialist, or The Team?

The decision as to whether each practitioner chooses to train in surgical and/or prosthodontic techniques or merely to refer patients, is of course down to the individual. However it is becoming clear that all practitioners will have a responsibility to offer patients this type of treatment if suitably indicated.

Consequently there is a clear need for all dental healthcare workers to familiarise themselves with the basic sciences that encompass endosseous dental implantology.

Whether simply offering patients the opportunity for referral, or indeed executing a treatment plan "in house", the future impact of implants on any individual clinic, is as great as its impact on the future of clinical dentistry *per se*.

Where to start?

The number of implant systems available on the market today could be as high as 70, however of these there are only seven which seem to dom-

Table I-1

Astra Tech Dental Implant System — Astra Tech AB, Mölndal, Sweden
Brånemark System™   Nobolpharma AD, Göteborg, Sweden
Core-Vent (Spectra) System — Dentsply®/Implant Division, California, USA
IMZ System — Friatec AG, Mannheim, Germany
Integral System — Calcitek®Inc, California, USA
ITI Implant System — Institute Straumann AG, Waldenburg, Switzerland
Steri-Oss System — Steri-Oss Inc, Anaheim, California, USA

Table I-1 Seven of the most commonly used implant systems.

Table I-2

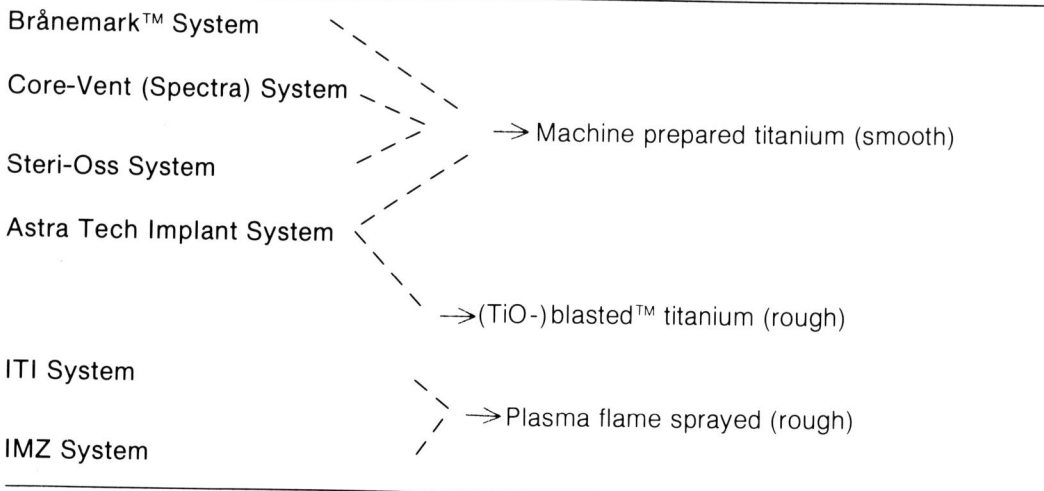

Table I-2 Types of titanium surface used in implant systems.

inate the global scene. These implants and their manufacturers are listed in table I-1.

The differing implant systems offer great diversity in their specifications, not least of which is the variety of biocompatible surfaces available for osseointegration. It is worth noting that the definition of osseointegration, which is based on a light microscope evaluation, is "... a direct structural and functional connection between ordered, living bone and the surface of a load-carrying implant."[8] Note that surface is not specified as being commercially pure (c.p.) titanium, and as such any material that can satisfy this definition at the light microscope level, can be considered osseointegrated.

Within the titanium implant range there appears to be three varieties of surface, giving either a smooth or rough finish (Table I-2). The other well documented biocompatible material being Hydroxyapatite, a crystalline structure of $Ca_{10}(PO_4)_6 OH_2$, which is usually coated on to a titanium implant.

Further diversity with regard to implant design only adds to the already confusing options. Clearly, only an adequate understanding of each system and what it can offer, will allow an informed decision. Many experienced implantologists today, utilise more than one implant system, to cater for the multitude of requirements from case to case.

The need for training!

It is necessary to stress continually, the need for adequate training prior to working with implants. Whilst within the scope of many practitioners, the placing of implants is a complex procedure which can not be achieved without relevant further studies.

Fortunately, a wide range of courses are available, run by implant companies, associations and individual practitioners who limit their practice to implants. Courses vary from basic science and system specific protocols, to advanced surgical and restorative techniques, ensuring that adequate opportunity exists for further study in the implant field.

It is hoped that this text will offer additional basic information, essential to be able to answer patients' questions pertaining to implants and to allow careful assessment and planning prior to referral and/or implant placement. It is worth bearing in mind that any implant case succeeds or fails as early as the evaluation stage, and the first chapter therefore addresses this important topic.

References

1 *Schnitman, P.A., Schulman, L.B.* Recommendations of the consensus development conference on dental implants. J Am Dent Assoc 1979; 98: 373-377.
2 *Adell, R., Lekholm, U., Rockler, B., Brånemark, P.-I.* A 15-year study of osseointegrated implants in the treatment of the edentulous jaw. Int J Oral Surg 1981; 10: 387-416.
3 *Hoogstraten, J., Lamers, L.M.* Patient satisfaction after insertion of an osseointegrated implant bridge. J Oral Rehab 1987; 14: 481-487.
4 *Akagawa, Y., Rachi, Y., Matsumoto, T., Tsuru, H.* Attitudes of removable denture patients toward dental implants. J Prosthet Dent 1988; 60: 362-363.
5 *Grogono, A.L., Lancaster, D.M., Finger, I.M.* Dental implants: A survey of patient's attitudes. J. Prosthet Dent 1989; 62: 573-576.
6 *Kiyak, H.A., Beach, B.H., Worthington, P., Taylor, T., Bolender, C., Evans, J.* The psychological impact of osseointegrated dental implants. Int J Oral Maxillofac Implants 1990; 5: 61-69.
7 *Blomberg, S., Lindquist, L.W.* Psychological reactions to edentulousness and treatment with jawbone-anchored bridges. Acta Psychiatr Scand 1983; 68: 251-262.
8 *Brånemark, P.-I.* Introduction to osseointegration. In: Tissue integrated prostheses. Osseointegration in clinical dentistry (eds *Brånemark, P.-I., Zarb, G., Albrektsson, T.*), p11. Berlin: Quintessence, 1985.

1 Patient Assessment and Radiographic Evaluation

The likelihood of patients walking through the door requesting treatment with, or asking for information on implants is clearly on the rise and many readers may already have come across such a request as a result of the increasing coverage of this topic in the media.

It is no longer acceptable to tell the patient that this is still experimental treatment, as this constitutes misleading advice. Such a request demands an evaluation of the situation based on a sound understanding of what can be achieved with dental implants.

It is often the case that patients are not suitable for treatment with implants, or that a conventional alternative may be preferable. A decision based on a thorough knowledge of the patient's medical and dental history, along with a full radiographic evaluation, will determine suitability. These areas will be covered in this chapter.

Initial consultation

At the initial consultation it is important to determine the patient's prime motivation for enquiring about implants[1]. As a cardinal rule it should be understood that aesthetics alone are NOT a good reason for seeking implants. It is likely that a new conventional bridge or indeed a more aesthetically pleasing denture, so long as it is functionally sound, will solve this problem at a fraction of the cost.

Function is the key complaint that should arouse your attention. A failing conventional bridge, the enduringly loose full denture, and the free end saddle (particularly unilateral) are classic scenarios which deserve consideration for rehabilitation with implants.

Psychologically based concerns also deserve attention, with caution. There are a number of interesting reasons that one can come across, for patients seeking implants. Such concerns often arise through sexual self awareness and/or embarrassment.

An example of this might be young patients who have lost anterior teeth which have been replaced with a partial denture due to the unrestored nature of the abutment teeth (which

15

MEDICAL HISTORY

GP's Name:

GP's Address: ....

....

1	Diabetes	11	Radiation
2	Hypertension	12	Steroids
3	Heart Disease	13	Allergies
4	Bleeding Diseases	14	Drug Sensitive
5	Lung Disease	15	Specify ....
6	GIT Disease	16	Epilepsy
7	Rheumatoid	17	Headaches
8	Osteoarthritis	18	Alcohol
9	Osteoporosis	19	Smoking
10	HIV/HBV Test	20	Other

21 Details of past history ....

....

....

22 Ongoing Medication

23 Patient's Signature ....

24 Surgeon's Signature ....

Fig 1-1 An appropriate dental card medical history.

Table 1-1   Contra Indications to Placement of Dental Implants

Absolute contra indications	Possible contra indications (Require further Investigation)
Uncontrolled diabetes	Systemic haematological disorders
Psychosis — unrealistic expectations, dysmorphophobia	Irradiation of jaws
	Liver and kidney disorders
Drug and alcohol abuse	Osteoporosis/low bone mineral content
Kidney dialysis	Local pathology
Pre-pubertal age	

their dentist would prefer not to prepare for fixed bridgework). This can lead to a loss of confidence due to the fact that their front teeth are "removable". Another example is the concerns of individuals who are unable to partake of intimate kissing etc., due to the embarrassing looseness of their dentures.

These very real concerns might be addressed successfully by dental implants, but it is often difficult to extract this kind of information from patients. Furthermore it is equally important that an understanding of the patient's expectations is clarified. A disproportionately high expectation represents one of the principal contra-indications and others have suggested that, should there be any doubt, a psychological assessment be sought.[1, 2]

A full medical history is required, and the use of a standard dental card history is inadequate. It only takes a short time to construct a full medical history sheet like that shown in figure 1-1, and this should be signed and stored with the patient's details. A list of contra-indications to treatment are given in table 1-1.

It should be understood that the placement of dental implants represents invasive dento-alveolar surgery. As such patients with stabilised cardiac disease should be prepared in the same way as all such patients for minor oral surgery, that is with appropriate antibiotic prophylaxis and consideration regarding the use of adrenaline based local anaesthetics. Clearly **there is no substitute for conferring with a patient's medical practitioner prior to surgery.** Surprisingly old age is not a contraindication, subject to good systemic and mental health but pre-pubertal youth does present problems due to the fact that implants are essentially ankylosed, and consequently they become submerged as skeletal alveolar growth progresses.

Osteoporosis is particularly relevant for the post menopausal woman, and it may be worthwhile seeking *Bone Mineral Content* evaluation as part of a routine *Bone Metabolic Counsel-*

ling procedure, especially if the patient is not on Hormone Replacement Therapy.[3]

The *dental history* will of course involve an oral examination, a radiographic examination, and a diagnostic evaluation using articulated study models.

The *oral examination* should take the form of a routine assessment of hard and soft tissues, of the oral and circum-oral structures. Do not assume that a clinically atrophic mandible infers that there is inadequate bone, this is rarely the case. Conversely a well formed maxilla may be mostly sinus cavitation. All clinical findings should therefore be considered in association with further investigations.

A *dental and periodontal evaluation* will elicit information on the presence of caries, periodontal disease, and oral hygiene status. It is of paramount importance that a patient be treated with any conventional dentistry indicated, since a sound dental status must exist prior to implant placement.

Soft tissues are further assessed for health and quality in terms of being keratinised or non-keratinised. The presence of non-keratinised tissue around an emerging abutment is not considered ideal, and may indicate the need for an autogenous gingival graft to increase the peri-implant zone of keratinised tissue.[4-7] An assessment of soft tissues should also determine their thickness. This can be done by measuring soft tissue thickness with a periodontal probe. It is then possible to map out the soft tissue thickness on a sectioned duplicate cast, thus highlighting residual ridge width (Fig 1-2). Alternatively bony ridge thickness can be measured directly using bone callipers.[8] This is referred to as *ridge mapping*.

Master study casts should be mounted and articulated, since an assessment of occlusal vertical dimension is necessary to determine the space available for the prosthetic superstructure. Furthermore, instructions should be given to the technician for a diagnostic wax-up to be fabricated (Fig 1-3), based on the proposed treatment plan. A useful hint is to ask the technician to place brass retention pins into the cast, to indicate the ideal position of the implants in relation to the diagnostic wax-up (Fig 1-4). The information and subsequent use of the diagnostic wax-up, reproduced as a surgical template (Fig 1-5) is discussed below.

In order to assess a case correctly, it is essential to undertake a full *radiographic evaluation*. As a minimum requirement an orthopantomograph (OPT) and intra-oral radiographs (IOR) are advised. The use of a Lateral Cephlogram (LC) is helpful in the edentulous case to determine lingual inclination of the atrophic mandible (Fig 1-6).

When planning for implants it is important to extract as much useful information as possible from your radiographs in order to aid in the evaluation and pre-surgical preparation.

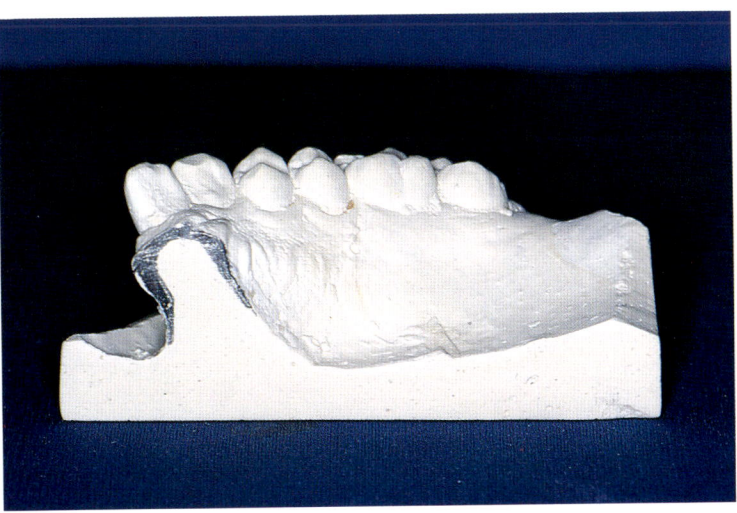

Fig 1-2 A diagnostic study model is sectioned and trimmed according to ridge mapping measurements, demonstrating the true alveolar ridge width available for implant placement.

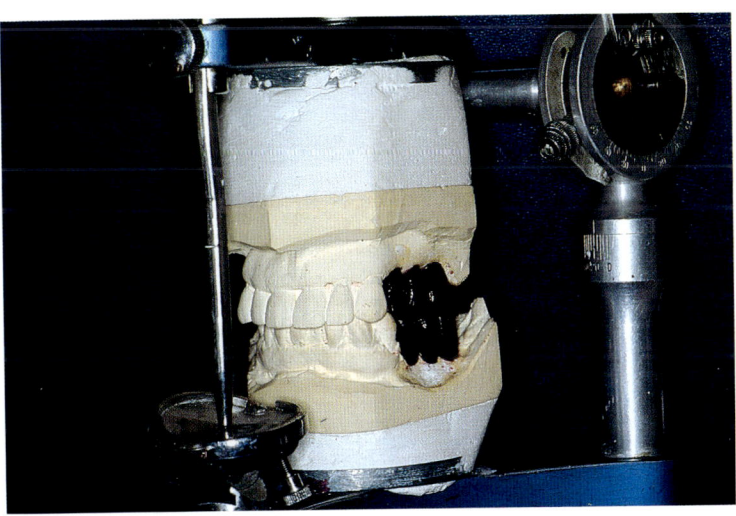

Fig 1-3 Articulated study models, provide useful information to aid treatment planning. A diagnostic wax-up further delineates the prosthetic, and hence surgical field, also providing vital information regarding occlusal form.

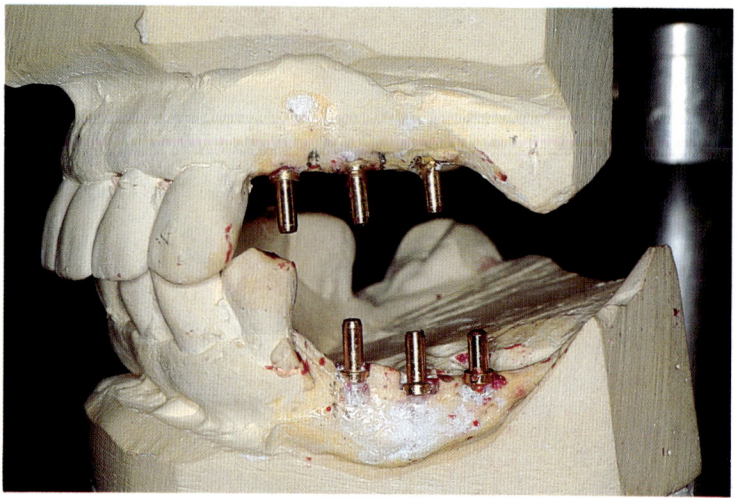

Fig 1-4 The use of brass retention pins, located in the study model, help support each unit of the diagnostic wax-up, and provide valuable visual information on the ideal mesio-distal positioning of the implants.

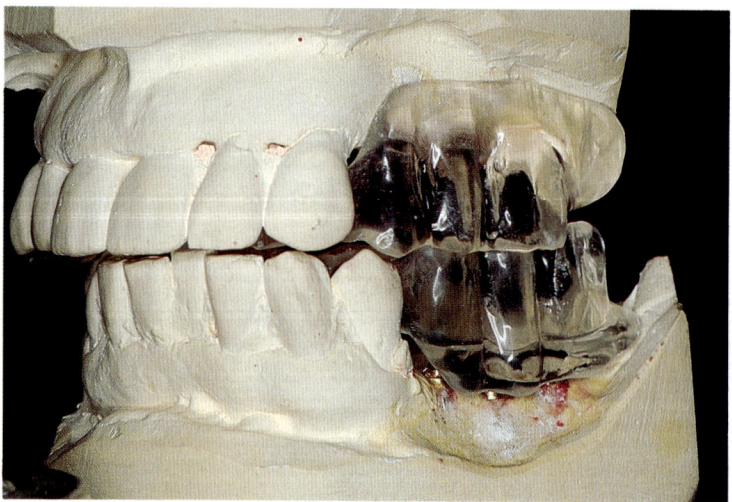

Fig 1-5 The diagnostic wax-up is conveniently reproduced in clear acrylic to act as a surgical template. This will ensure accurate positioning of the implants during the surgical procedure.

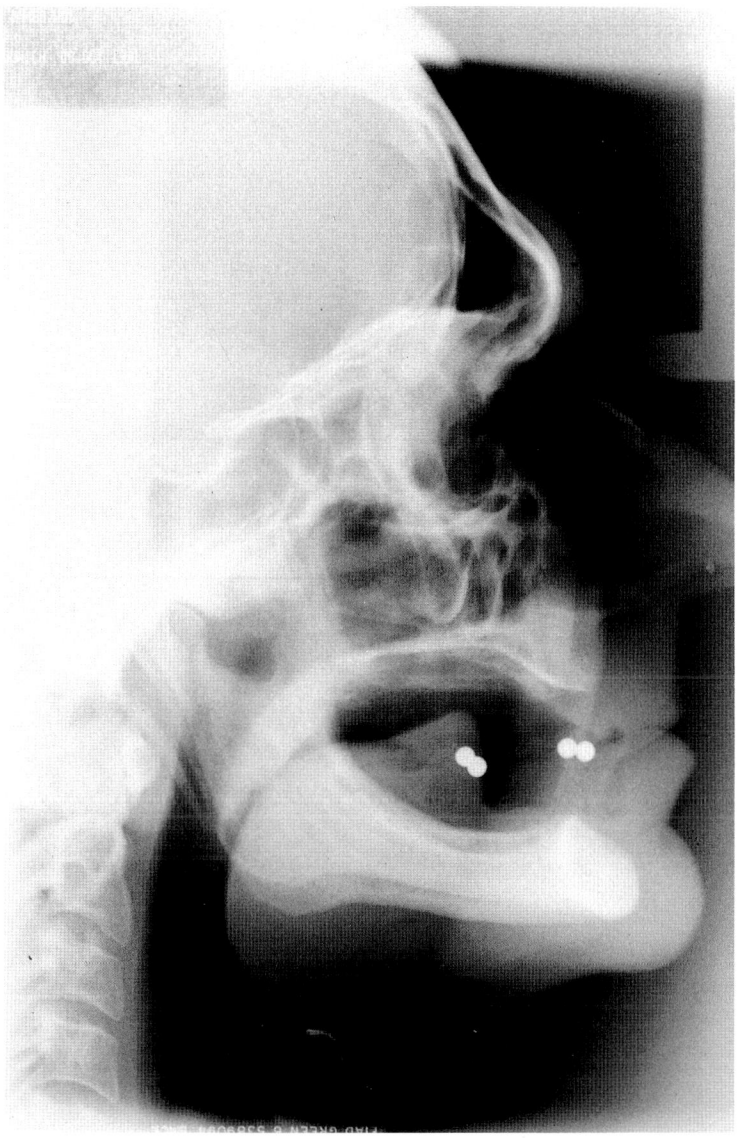

Fig 1-6 For the edentulous patient a lateral cephalogram allows an assessment of the pattern of resorption, highlighting the degree of mandibular lingual inclination. The use of ball bearings also allows an assessment of the relative position of the incisal edge to the crest of the ridge.

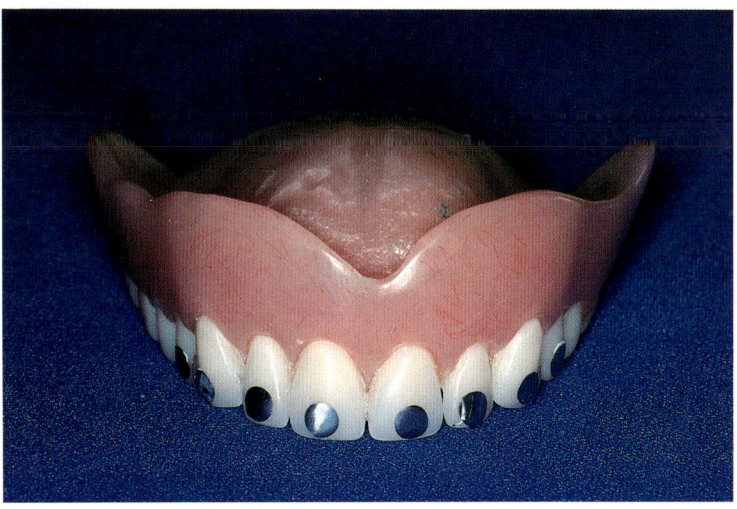

Fig 1-7 Foil spots, of a defined size, are punched out of the foil of a periapical film and stuck to the surface of each tooth, on the patient's denture, thus relating their position to the OPT, and providing information regarding variable distortion.

If measurements for bone height are to be deduced from such radiographs, it is necessary to always place a radiographic marker, such as a ball bearing, in the planned operative field; this will allow you to determine distortion. An average OPT machine will give a distortion factor of between 20-40% magnification, depending on the age of the machine. Dividing the measured bone height by this factor will give an accurate estimate of true bone height (TBH) available.

In order to define the surgical field, it is useful to place a radiopaque stent in the patient's mouth. For the denture wearer, it is possible to place foil spots on each tooth of the denture (Fig 1-7), so as to transfer tooth position to the radiograph (Fig 1-8). For partially dentate cases, the *diagnostic wax-up* is essential (Figs 1-9 & 1-10), and it is useful to have a suck down splint produced over a cast of such wax-ups which can then be placed in the mouth prior to taking the OPT (Fig 1-11). The use of Barium Sulphate powder (Fig 1-12), painted on the surface of the splint will demonstrate the position of the teeth satisfactorily.

Highlighting in soft pencil, vital structures on the radiograph, such as inferior dental nerves, ridge crests, nasal floor, sinuses, and adjacent teeth will clearly demonstrate the confines of the surgical field. It is now

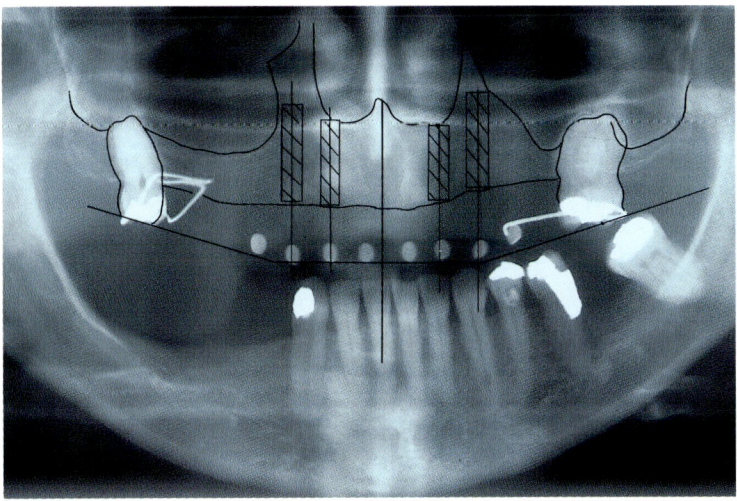

Fig 1-8 The position of each denture tooth is clearly transferred to the OPT as individual radiopaque spots. The position of each implant is drawn in pencil on the radiograph to coincide with these markers.

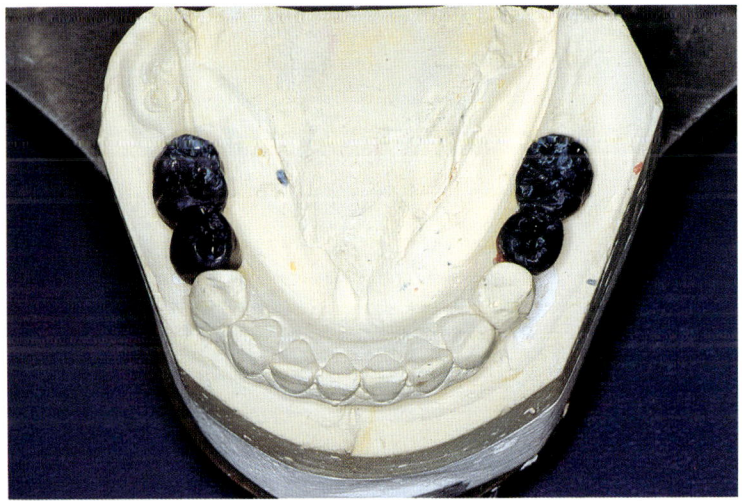

Fig 1-9 A Kennedy class I mandibular case is provisionally assessed with bilateral diagnostic wax-ups to restore the free end saddles. Diagnostic wax-ups should provide accurate information on occlusal table width, buccolingual form, and the mesiodistal position of each dental unit.

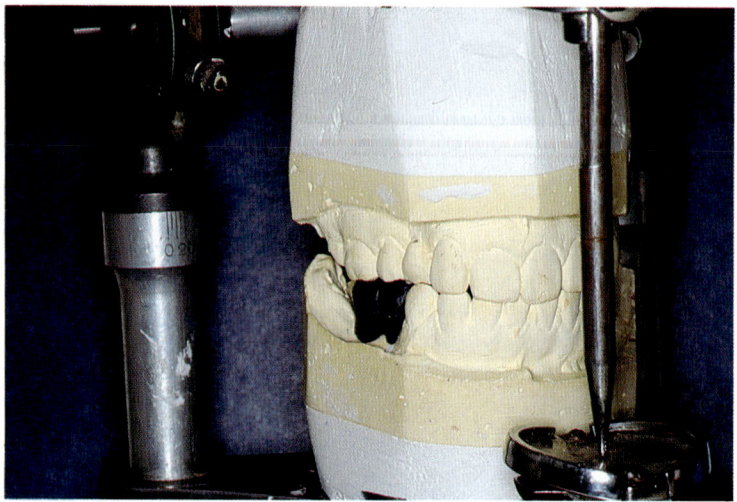

Fig 1-10 Study models are mounted on a semi-adjustable articulator, to allow assessment of occlusal function on both working and non-working sides.

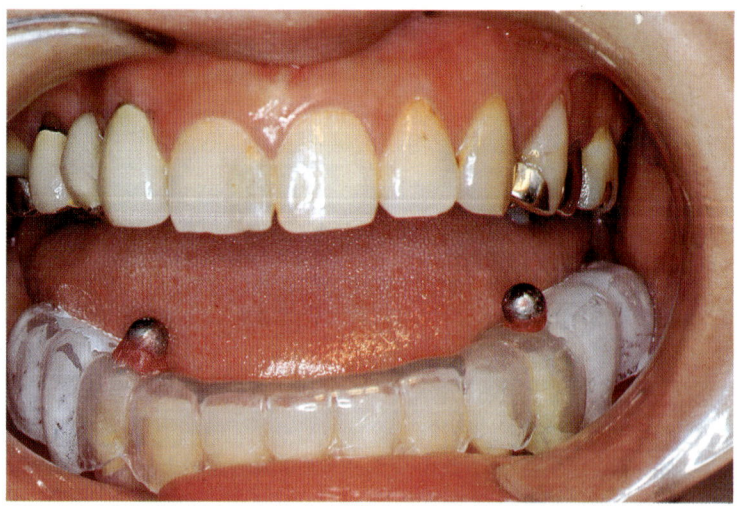

Fig 1-11 A suck down splint is manufactured over a solid cast duplicate of the diagnostic wax-ups. For the partially dentate patient this is a useful template since it benefits from tooth borne support, and is not displaced during surgery. For diagnostic radiographs, additional information can be sought by providing radiographic markers such as ball bearings.

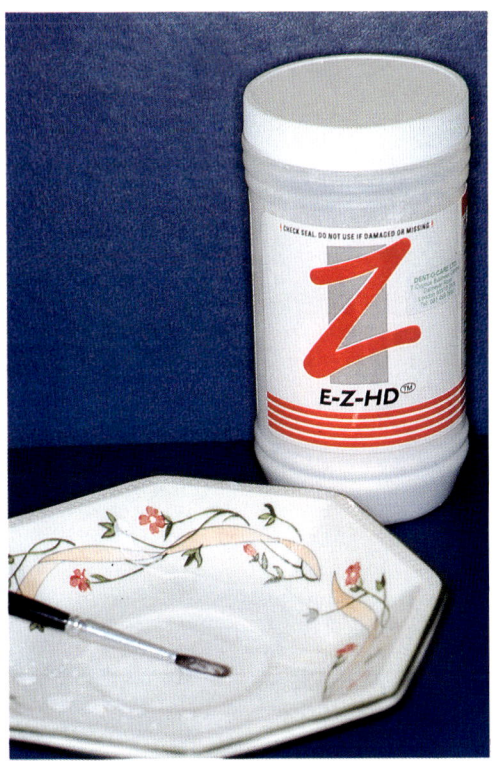

Fig 1-12 The use of Barium Sulphate painted on to the surface of the template is another method that allows the transfer of tooth position to the diagnostic radiograph, thus confirming the mesio-distal position of each dental unit.

possible to superimpose the shape of the implants, using a pre-magnified radiographic template (Fig 1-13), and to determine both position and length of implants from the information provided (Fig 1-14).

This is a useful exercise to do in front of the patient as it gives valuable insight into the treatment plan and often stimulates the right kind of questions. Tied in with the diagnostic wax-up, this leaves the patient in little doubt about treatment aims and aspirations. The splint can now be stored for use at a later date as a surgical template during implant insertion. This will ensure accurate positioning of implants in the mesio-distal, axial, and bucco-lingual relations, as indicated on the diagnostic radiograph and study models.

When faced with potential complications, such as thin ridges or implants placed over the inferior dental nerves, it is often considered advisable to arrange for a *Computed Tomography Scan* (CT scans).[9-13] The CT scan is able to provide information in three dimensions, with insignificant distortion (Fig 1-15, 1-16). As such it is possible to determine ridge width and the amount of avail-

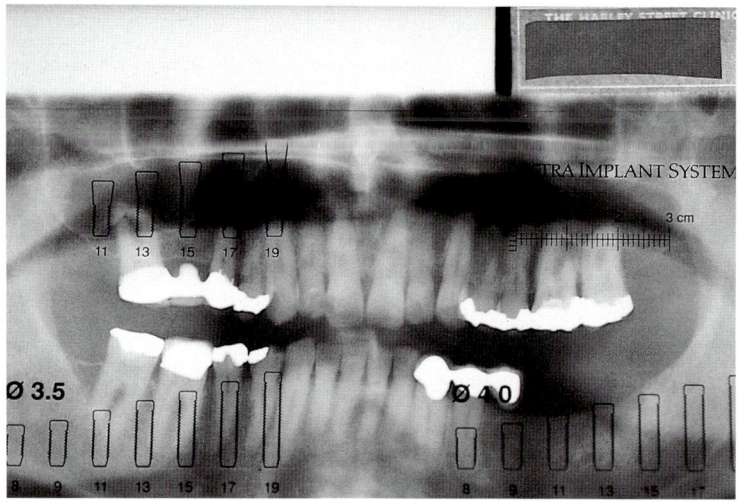

Fig 1-13 Some implant companies provide clear radiographic fixture guides (Astra Tech AB, Mölndal, Sweden) for differing degrees of distortion. These can be used to trace the position of an implant on to a radiograph itself or a tracing of the radiograph.

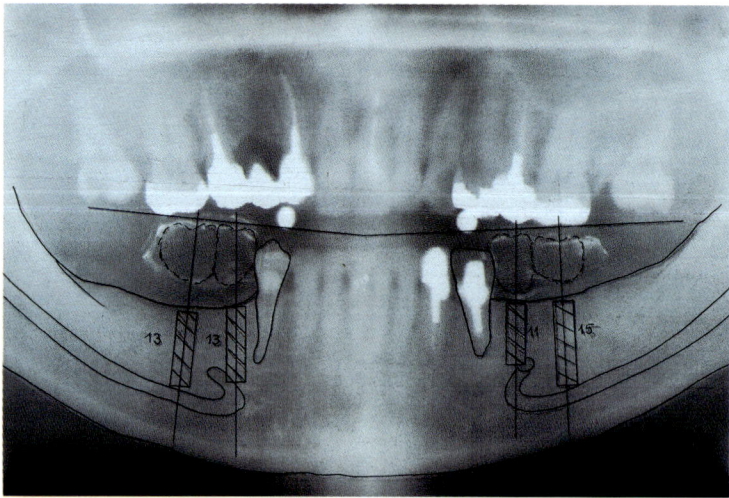

Fig 1-14 The diagnostic OPT can be used to highlight the surgical field, the mesio-distal position of each implant to be placed, and their relation to any vital structures. It is of paramount importance that an assessment of distortion is made and that the relative fixture guide is chosen to relate the correct implant dimensions to the radiograph (see Fig 1-11).

26

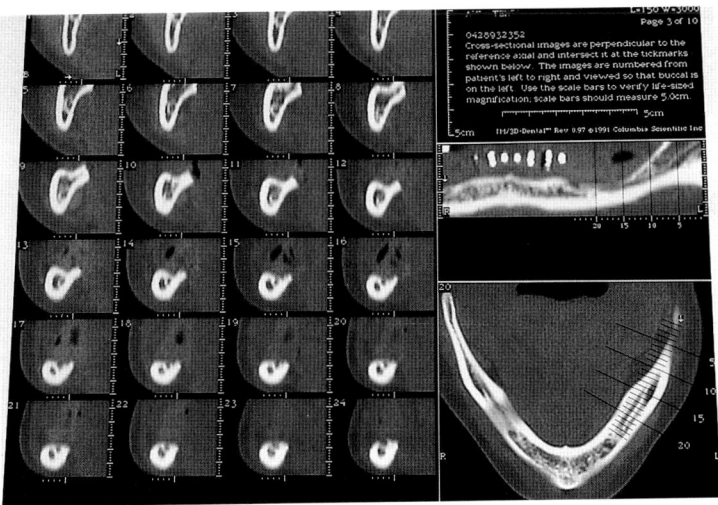

Fig 1-15 The use of CT scans may be essential when implants are to be placed close to vital structures, or where conventional radiographs fail to provide the desired information. Specific software (3D/Dental software, Columbia Scientific Incorporated, Columbia, MD) is available to allow high quality images in, *transverse section*, panoramic views and 3 Dimensions.

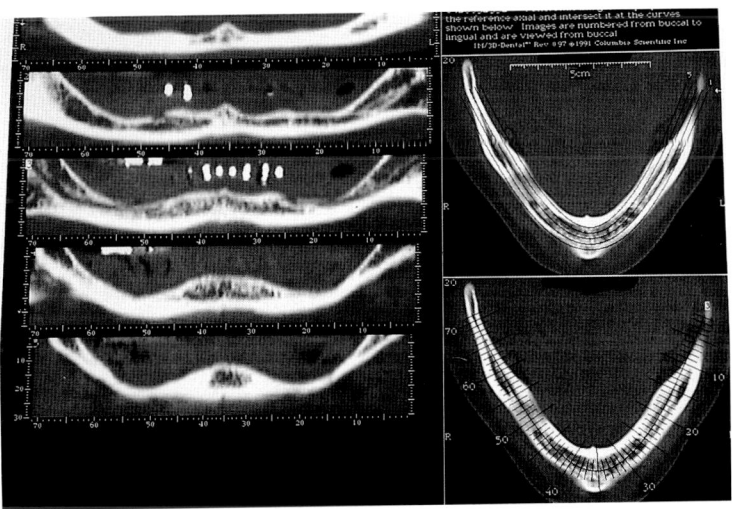

Fig 1-16 The use of CT scans may be essential when implants are to be placed close to vital structures, or where conventional radiographs fail to provide the desired information. Specific software (3D/Dental software, Columbia Scientific Incorporated, Columbia, MD) is available to allow high quality images in transverse section *panoramic views* and 3 Dimensions.

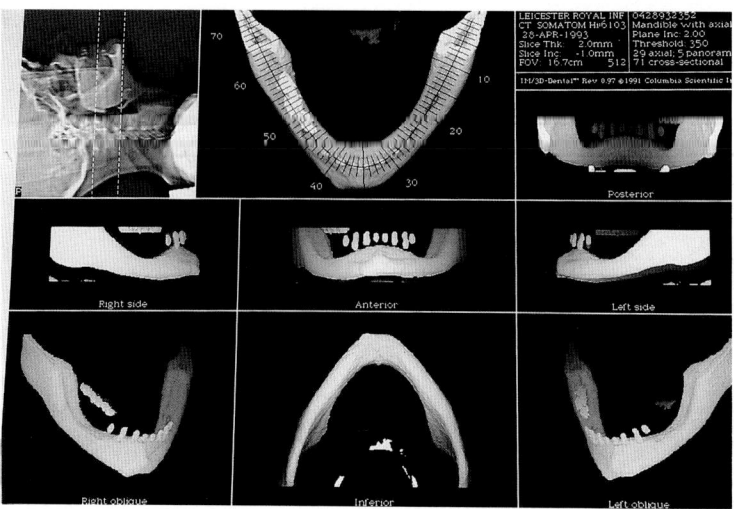

Fig 1-17 The use of CT scans may be essential when implants are to be placed close to vital structures, or where conventional radiographs fail to provide the desired information. Specific software (3D/Dental software, Columbia Scientific Incorporated, Columbia, MD) is available to allow high quality images in transverse section, panoramic views and *3 Dimensions.*

able bone around vital structures with greater accuracy.

It is also possible to build a 3-D picture of the underlying bony morphology,[14] which can help in pre-planning of surgery (Fig 1-17). However CT scans are expensive, and can cause some concern to the patient, who may need to lay motionless for as much as twenty minutes while the scan is taken. It is also important to weigh up risk versus benefit in respect of radiation dosage which may vary from scanner to scanner, particularly in the light of other techniques described, which may allow the accurate placement of implants adjacent to vital structures

using conventional dental radiographic techniques.[15]

When referring cases to a surgeon it is often useful to classify ridge morphology on the basis of degrees of atrophy. In implantology the most commonly quoted classification is that proposed by Lekholm and Zarb,[16] which also gives an indication of bone quality (Fig 1-18, 1-19). Other more complex but accurate classifications are also occasionally utilised.[17]

Having completed your assessment and confirmed patient suitability it is advisable to send the patient away with an instruction booklet, which should describe in full detail all the

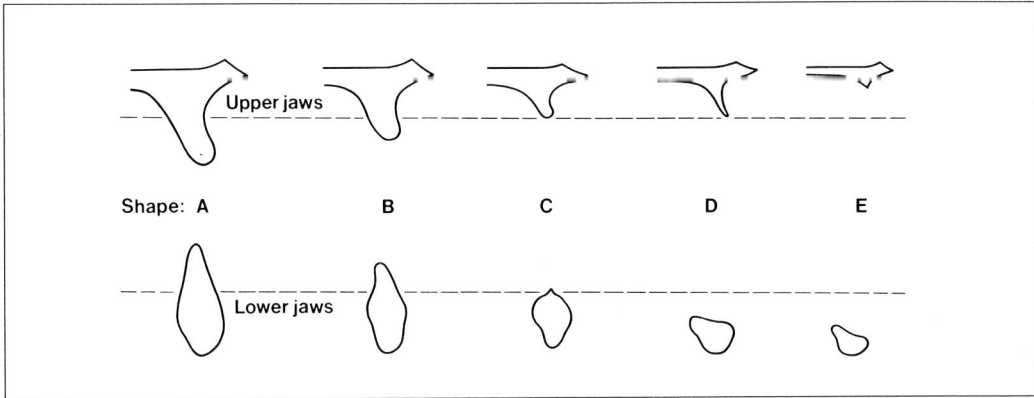

Fig 1-18 Classification for residual ridge morphology as proposed by Lekholm & Zarb: (A) most of the alveolar ridge is present; (B) moderate residual ridge resorption has occurred; (C) advanced residual ridge resorption has occurred and only basal bone remains; (D) some resorption of the basal bone has started; (E) extreme resorption of the basal bone has taken place.

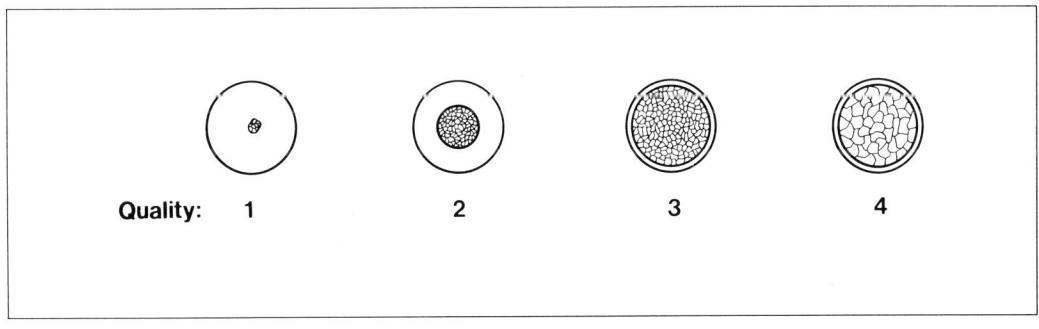

Fig 1-19 Classification of jawbone quality as proposed by Lekholm & Zarb: (1) almost the entire jaw is composed of homogenous compact bone; (2) a thick layer of compact bone surrounds a core of dense trabecular bone; (3) a thin layer of compact bone surrounds a core of dense trabecular bone of favourable strength; (4) a thin layer of cortical bone surrounds a core of low density trabecular bone.

possible ramifications of implant surgery, and how the treatment is likely to proceed.

An opportunity for patients to raise questions before final consultation is essential, allowing those last minute concerns to be discussed and hopefully quelled.

Final consultation should be arranged no more than one week prior to surgery. This ensures that all final discussions are fresh in the mind of both you and your patient.

At this consultation it is often desirable to have a third party present, preferably next-of-kin, so that there are no misunderstandings. Should it be decided to employ sedation or a general anaesthetic this is also a good opportunity to confirm arrangements for escort, and to discuss post operative care.

The use of consent forms is strongly indicated, and should cover consent for surgery and any anaesthetic procedure, as well as highlighting the patient's understanding of possible complications.

The value of consent will vary depending on its structure and the medicolegal requirements of each individual country. The safest recommendation is that you consult with your professional indemnity society, and seek their advice on this matter.

References

1 *Laney, W.R.* Selecting edentulous patients for tissue-integrated prostheses. Int J Oral Maxillofac Implants 1986; 1: 129-138.

2 *Blomberg, S., Lindquist, L.W.* Psychological reactions to edentulousness and treatment with jawbone-anchored bridges. Acta Psychiatr Scand 1983; 68: 251-262.

3 *Roberts, W.E., Simmons, K.E., Garetto, L.P., DeCastro, R.A.* Bone physiology and metabolism in dental implantology: Risk factors for osteoporosis and other metabolic bone diseases. Implant Dent 1992; 1: 11-21.

4 *Rapley, J.W., Mills, M.P., Wylam, J.* Soft tissue management during implant maintenance. Int J Periodont Rest Dent 1992; 12: 373-381.

5 *Hangorsky, U., Bissada, N.F.* Clinical assessment of free gingival graft effectiveness on the maintenance of periodontal health. J Periodontol 1980; 51: 274-278.

6 *Wennstrom, J.L., Lindhe, J.* Plaque-induced gingival inflammation in the absence of attached gingiva in dogs. J Clin Periodontol 1983; 10: 266-276.

7 *van Steenberghe, D.* Periodontal aspects of osseointegrated oral implants ad modum Brånemark. Dent Clin North Am 1988; 32: 355-370.

8 *Wilson, D.J.* Ridge mapping for determination of alveolar ridge width. Int J Oral Maxillofac implants 1989; 4: 41-43.

9 *Schwarz, M.S., Rothman, S.L.G., Rhodes, M.L., Chafetz, N.* Computed tomography: Part 1. Preoperative assessment of the mandible for endosseous implant surgery. J Oral Maxillofac Implants 1987; 2: 137-141.

10 *Schwarz, M.S., Rothman, S.L.G., Rhodes, M.L., Chafetz, N.* Computed tomography: Part 2. Preoperative assessment of the maxilla for endosseous implant surgery. Int J Oral Maxillofac Implants 1987; 2: 143-148.

11 *Williams, M.Y.A., Mealey, B.L., Hallmon, W.W.* The role of computerized tomography in dental implantology. Int J Oral Maxillofac Implants 1992; 7: 373-380.

12 *McGivney, G.P., Haughton, V., Stradt, J.A., Eichholz, J.E., Lubar, D.M.* A comparison of computer assisted tomography and data-gathering modalities in prosthodontics. Int J Oral Maxillofac Implants 1986; 1: 55-56.

13 *Quirynen, M., Lamoral, Y., Dekeyser, C., Peene, P., van Steenberghe, D., Bonte, J., Baert, A.L.* The CT Scan standard reconstruction technique for reliable jaw bone volume determination. Int J Oral Maxillofac Implants 1990; 5: 384-389.

14 *Kraut, R.A.* Utilization of 3D/dental software for precise implant site selection: Clinical reports. Implant Dent 1992; 1: 134-140.

15 *Gelb, D.A.* Gelb depth gauge: A diagnostic aid in implant placement. Int J Peridont Rest Dent 1992; 12: 301-309.

16 *Lekholm, U., Zarb, G.A.* Patient selection and preparation. In: Tissue integrated prostheses. Osseointegration in clinical dentistry (eds *Brånemark, P.-I., Zarb, G., Albrektsson, T.*), pp 201-209. Berlin: Quintessence, 1985.

17 *Cawood, J.I., Howell, R.A.* A classification of the edentulous jaws. Int J Oral Maxillofac Surg 1988; 17: 232-236.

2 Surgical Placement of Implants

Results of a 15-year study on Bråne-mark implants, published by Adell et al in 1981,[1] included details of a definitive surgical procedure essential to the long term viability of the osseointegrated implant. This procedure, which previous articles had identified as encouraging an intimate connection between an implant, of defined geometry and surface preparation, with living bone[2-4] remains the key to a predictable osseointegration technique.

With implant manufacturers presenting fixtures of varying specification, the surgical protocol varies to allow for design specificity. By way of an example, the preparation for a hollow basket implant requires the use of a trephine drill rather than a solid drill. However, a common theme that exists throughout, is the aim to inflict minimal physical and thermal trauma to vital osseous tissues and to encourage close apposition of the fixture to bone for effective primary fixation. A surgical protocol that breaches this theme will likely result in a fibrous encapsulation of the implant, which is then less able to withstand biomechanical and microbial insult.[5, 6]

The importance of minimal heat production during bone preparation has been highlighted by Eriksson, whose thesis[7] and subsequent publications[8-10] established a threshold temperature of 47°C for one minute, if bone was not to be irreversibly damaged. Implant companies have endeavoured to design drills that impart minimal heat through cutting, introducing concepts of internal and external irrigation. Research has failed to show any significant advantage between the techniques[11, 12] but emphasises the need for an efficient supply of copious saline irrigation. This would suggest that the most important piece of equipment is the drill unit which should allow low cutting speeds, with a facility to pump saline directly onto or through the drill.

The surgical protocol presented below, which aims to reflect the nature of this general theme, is specific to the Astra Tech Implant System (Astra Tech AB, Mölndal, Sweden). It will be used throughout this text since this is the system used by the author. An effort will be made to point out variations that may occur with other implant systems, but this chapter is not intended to be a definitive source for the surgical protocol. The reader is encouraged to seek a more detailed protocol from the specific manufacturer of the implant system of their choice.

General Surgical Protocol

As part of the routine pre-operative requirements, all patients are given prophylactic antibiotics of choice and are asked to rinse out their mouth with 0.2% w/v chlorhexidine mouthwash (Corsodyl-SmithKline Beecham Ltd, Brentford, UK) for one minute.

There may be a need to establish an anaesthetic protocol for patients who request that they be unconscious during surgery. Sedation by intravenous titration of 10-15mg of Midazolam (Hypnovel®, Roche Products Ltd, England) or a similar anxiolytic is often sufficient to sustain a peaceful response and a degree of short acting amnesia. The option of a general anaesthetic should only be considered in advanced surgical cases, since this is essentially a minor operative procedure. It is important that prior consent always be obtained and that an appropriately trained clinician be responsible for the anaesthetic induction and maintenance.

Local anaesthetic (Xylocaine-Adrenaline 2%, Astra AB, Södertälje, Sweden) is administered via infiltration and/or regional blocks, accord-

ing to the surgical requirement.

In working towards a sterile environment, it is required that the patient should be swabbed with 0.1% w/v chlorhexidine and then draped. Both surgeon and nurse should scrub and gown up, making sure that the surgical gloves are non powdered since this may contaminate the implant surface (Fig 2-1). It is useful to have an unscrubbed runner, to avoid unnecessary contact with non sterile items.

The *incision* is normally placed either in the buccal sulcus so that the line of incision is distant from the surgical site, or is placed along the crest of the ridge (Fig 2-2), which facilitates surgical access, and reduces post-operative haematoma. However a crestal incision may increase the risk of implant fenestration, with subsequent infection. It may be that the ideal solution is a paracrestal incision offset to the palatal or lingual side.

In raising the flap it is essential that a sound mucoperiosteum is stripped from the bone (Fig 2-3) with limited exposure of the underlying alveolus, allowing an appreciation of ridge contours, particularly buccal and lingual concavities. Excessive damage to the periosteal lining will likely result in marginal bone resorption around the implants with soft tissue downgrowth which may compromise osseointegration. The use of high quality, sharp surgical instruments is to be commended.

Clearly an awareness of the surgical field, anatomical boundaries such as

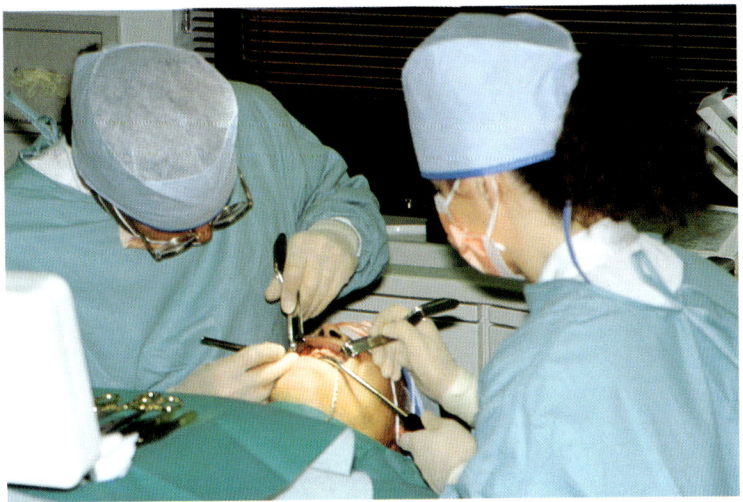

Fig 2-1 Surgical Protocol requires that an aseptic technique should be employed when placing dental implants.

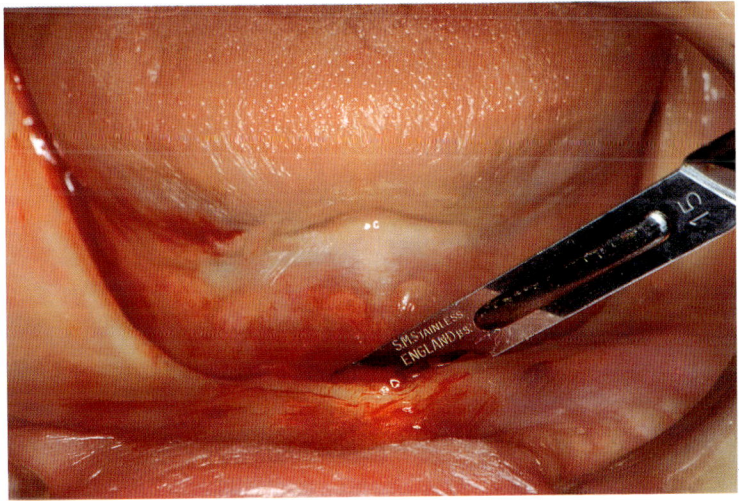

Fig 2-2 The incision is placed according to the surgeon's preference. In the case shown, the incision has been placed lingually to avoid direct trauma to the superficial inferior alveolar nerve.

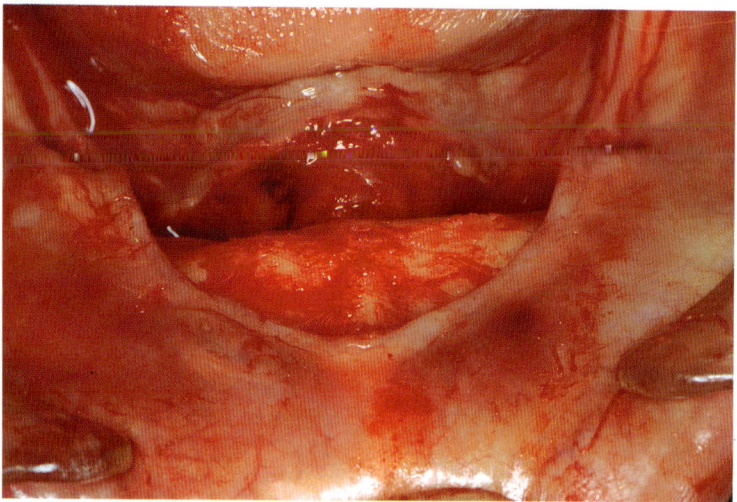

Fig 2-3 A sound mucoperiosteum is raised, with limited elevation that should provide adequate visual and instrument access. Over stripping of the periosteum will delay healing and may compromise bone vitality.

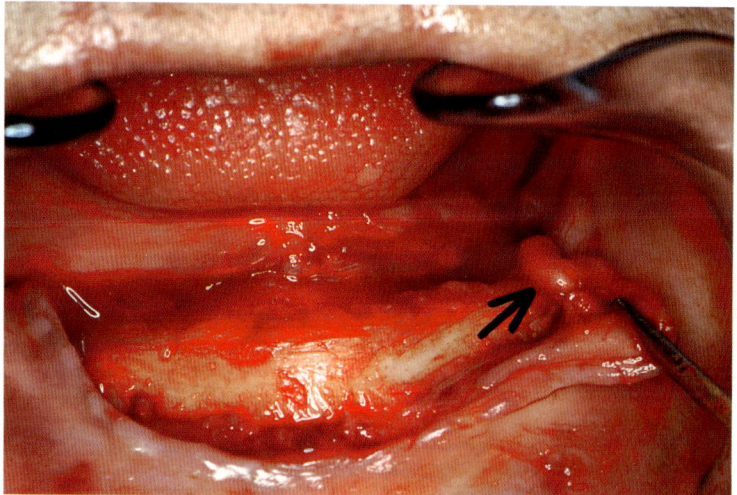

Fig 2-4 When placing mandibular implants it is necessary to carry out blunt dissection to localise and isolate the neurovascular bundles (arrow), as they emerge from the mental foramen or superficial canal.

floor of nose or antrum and knowledge of vital structures is essential. In the mandible, it is necessary to carry out blunt subperiosteal dissection to locate the exiting neurovascular bundle from the mental foramen (Fig 2-4) in order to avoid traumatising this vital structure. Identification of the nasopalatine neurovascular bundle is also necessary when placing implants in the premaxilla. A breach of anatomical boundaries or an encroachment of vital structures without forethought, will likely result in implant failure, or complications such as paraesthesia or anaesthesia of the mental nerve distribution. There is a clear need to be aware of the anatomy of any surgical field even if simply assessing the case for referral and the reader is encouraged to pursue a refresher course on this subject.

In light of the above, it would be prudent to approach the placement of implants in the posterior maxilla and mandible with caution, since damage to the maxillary antra and the inferior dental nerve are to be avoided. Notwithstanding this statement, it is imperative that an adequately trained surgeon should utilise all available clinical and radiographic data to ensure a margin of safety when implants are utilised in the posterior regions.

Prior to surgical preparation of the bone for implant insertion, it may be necessary to alter the morphology of the crestal bone, reducing any "knife edge" ridge and creating an even contour with an adequate bone width. This will depend on the width of implant to be used. The use of bone files is perhaps preferable to the large bone burs, since they offer greater control over ridge reduction and allow the early harvesting of autogenous bone, which may be of value for grafting purposes, later in the procedure (Fig 2-5).

The surgical template is now placed in situ (Fig 2-6), ensuring that it is correctly seated. In the partially dentate patient the template should always be tooth borne so that the seating is not interfered with by soft tissue flaps.

In order to prepare implant sites in the host bone, efficiently and atraumatically, it is essential to use the recommended instrumentation (Fig 2-7). It is wise for all members of staff to familiarise themselves with this instrumentation and be aware of handling and storage instructions which will vary between manufacturers. *The improper handling of instrumentation may well compromise surgical success.*

Common to all systems is the gradual preparation of implant sites with a series of drills which increase in width (Fig 2-8), and which are used at speeds ranging from 500-2000 rpm under copious saline irrigation. The first of these drilling steps is the *guide drill*, a small rosehead bur used to pierce the outer cortex, marking the implant site for preparation (Fig 2-9), as indicated by the surgical stent. It is at this early stage that the surgeon first appreciates the true nature of bony quality.

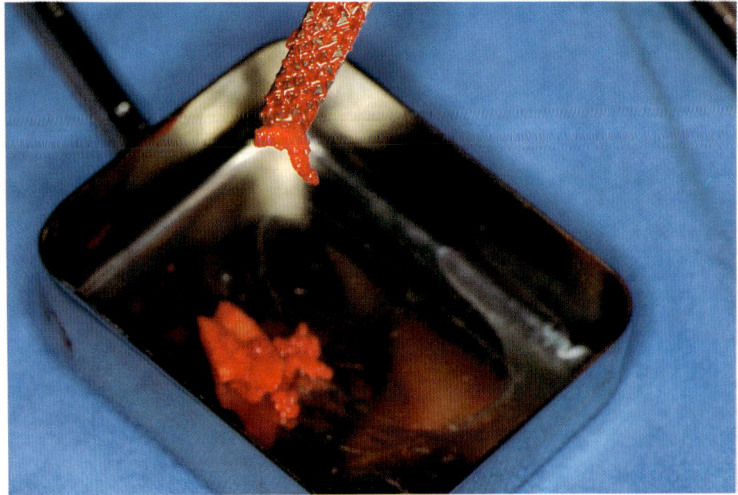

Fig 2-5 The knife-edged ridge will always require either augmentation or reduction to create adequate crestal bone to circumscribe the fixture. In reducing the ridge the use of a bone file is effective and allows the bone chips to be harvested for future use, if indicated.

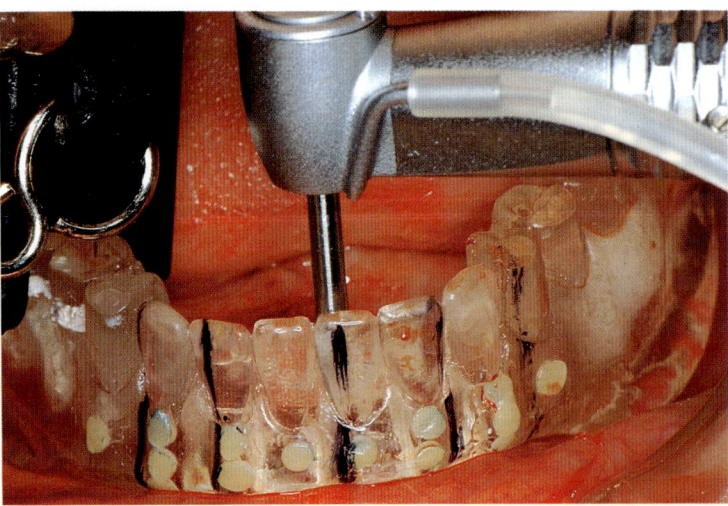

Fig 2-6 To ensure that the implants are positioned in a manner that relates to the final prosthesis, it is essential to use a surgical template (stent) to guide the preparation of fixture sites.

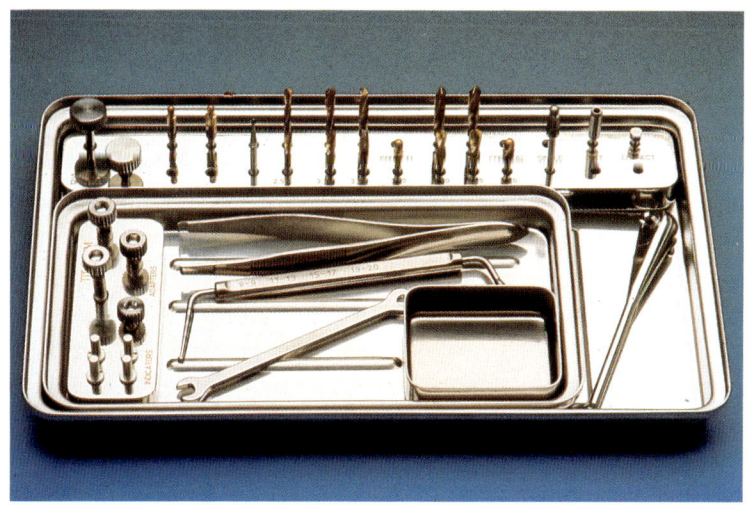

Fig 2-7 All implant manufacturers recommend that only approved instrumentation be used to guarantee precise and atraumatic preparation of the fixture sites.

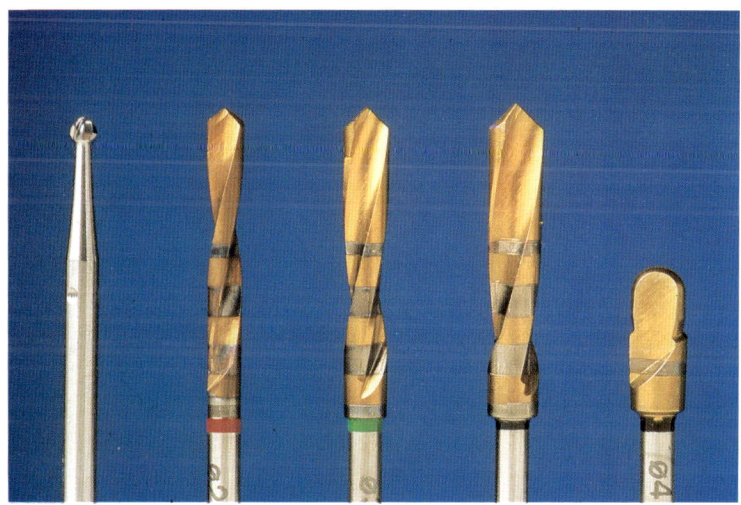

Fig 2-8 The Astra Tech Tiger™ Drills are laser banded to correspond to available implant lengths allowing easy assessment of preparation depth and are available in a range of widths and lengths to aid precise preparation.

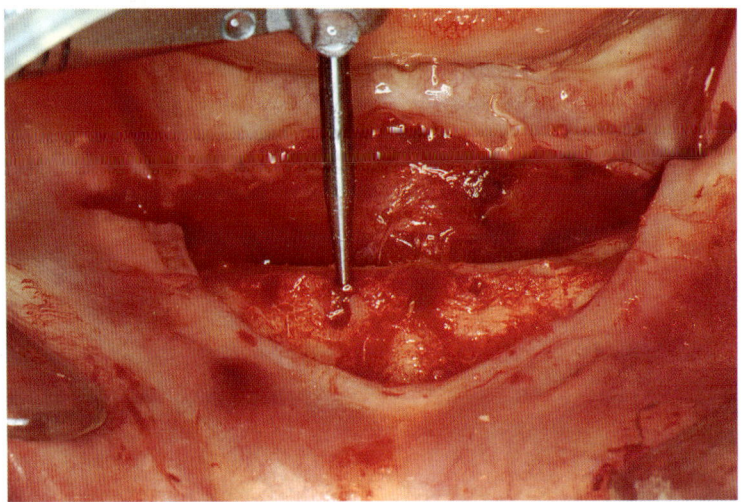

Fig 2-9 The rosehead bur or guide drill is used to perforate the outer cortex thus indicating implant position. It also provides the surgeon with an opportunity to assess bone quality.

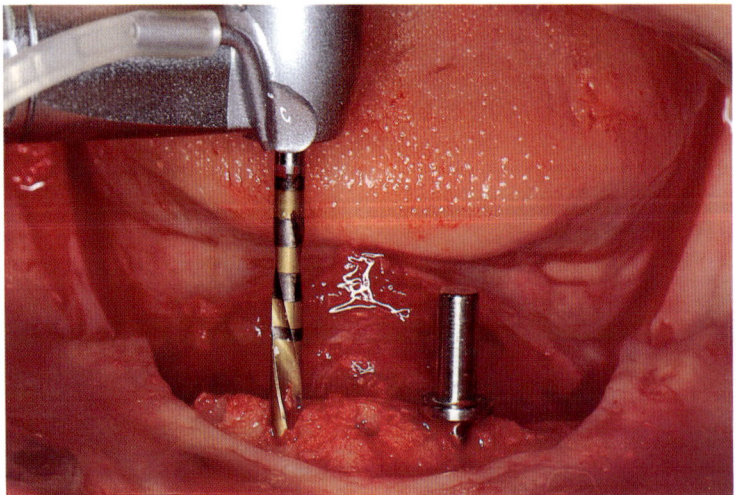

Fig 2-10 Preparation of the fixture sites will determine implant angulation and inclination. Control over fixture positioning and their relationship to one another is aided by the use of direction indicators.

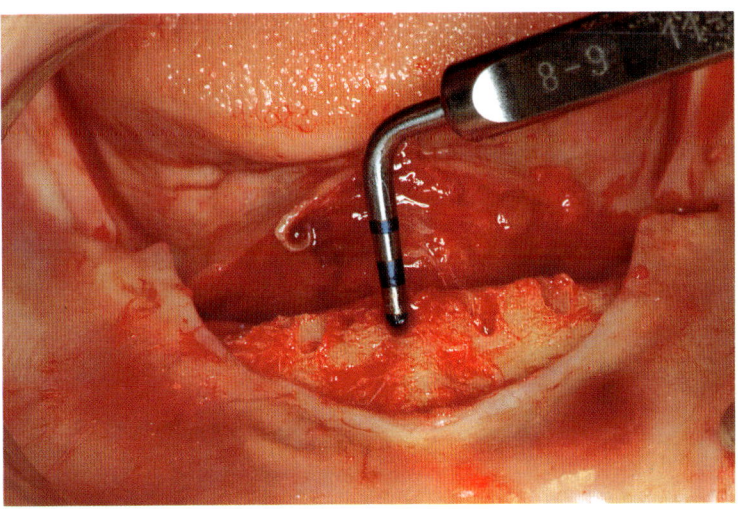

Fig 2-11 Preparation depth can be confirmed by use of a depth gauge, which in this case utilises the same laser bands as on the Tiger™ Drills.

Subsequent drilling steps will determine implant length, position and inclination. The relative position of one implant to another may have considerable bearing on the prosthetic reconstruction and all systems recommend the use of direction indicators to help in judging the ideal relation of one implant to another (Fig 2-10). If using a self tapping implant it should be possible, having assessed bone quality, to select the appropriate final preparation width to provide optimal primary fixation. In contrast, the preparation of bone for press fit or non self tapping implants requires a definitive preparation width, regardless of bone quality. The use of trephines, canon drills, or twist drills will depend on implant design, but all systems provide a measuring facility to ensure accuracy of preparation depth (Fig 2-11), and a range of drills to select appropriate preparation width.

The design of a drill should encourage maximum bone cutting efficiency at low speeds and should ensure that saline irrigation is directed to the tip of the drill, where control of heat production is critical (Fig 2-12). Ideally the drill should encourage the flushing out or collection of bone debris which not only leaves a patent preparation, but if harvested as autogenous bone mush can be used as bone grafting material, if required at a later stage (Fig 2-13).

For the standard Astra implant shown in Fig 2-14 there are no further preparatory drilling steps, as the

41

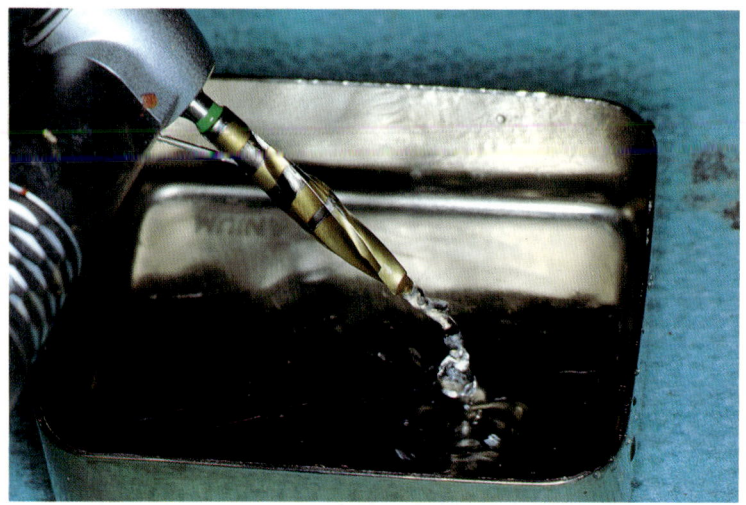

Fig 2-12 Whether using internal or external irrigation, the drill design and saline distribution should predictably direct maximum irrigation to the cutting tip, which is most at risk of causing thermal trauma to surrounding bone.

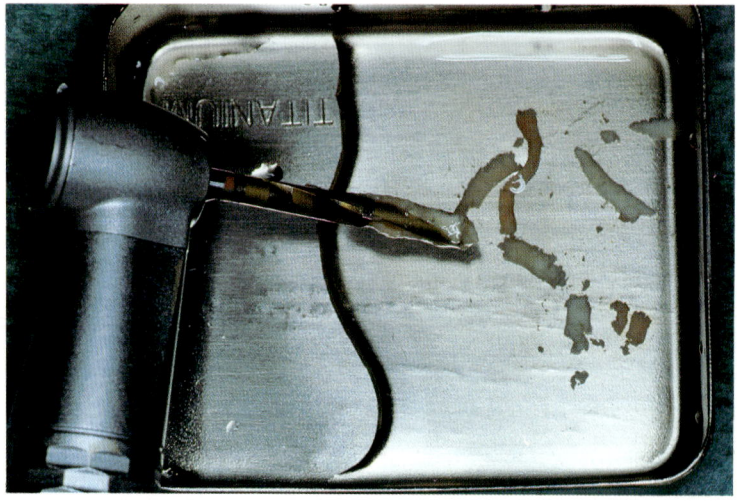

Fig 2-13 The drill should encourage complete removal of bone debris from the preparation site. Ideally such bone should be removed in a way that it can be harvested for future use, if indicated, as autogenous bone graft.

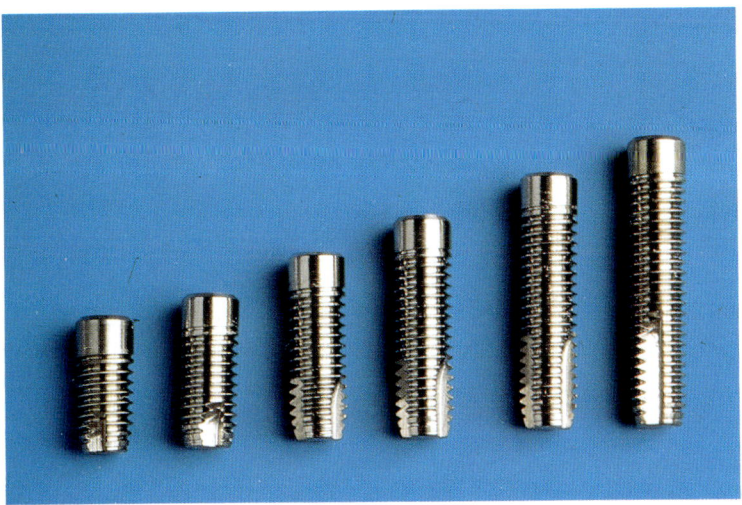

Fig 2-14 The standard Astra Tech Dental Implant is a self tapping titanium fixture, which is available in seven lengths, 8, 9, 11, 13, 15, 17, 19mm (only six lengths shown) and two diameters 3.5 and 4.0mm (3.5mm diameter pictured).

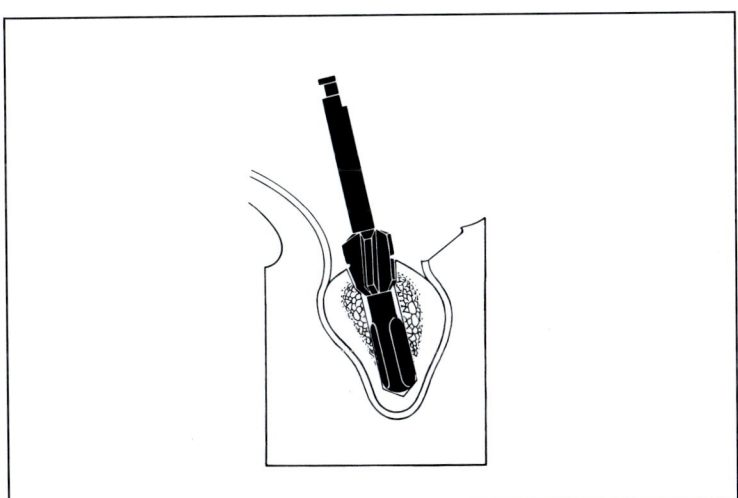

Fig 2-15 The countersink preparation removes additional crestal bone in order that the fixture site is able to receive the head of an implant which may, by design, be wider than the implant body.

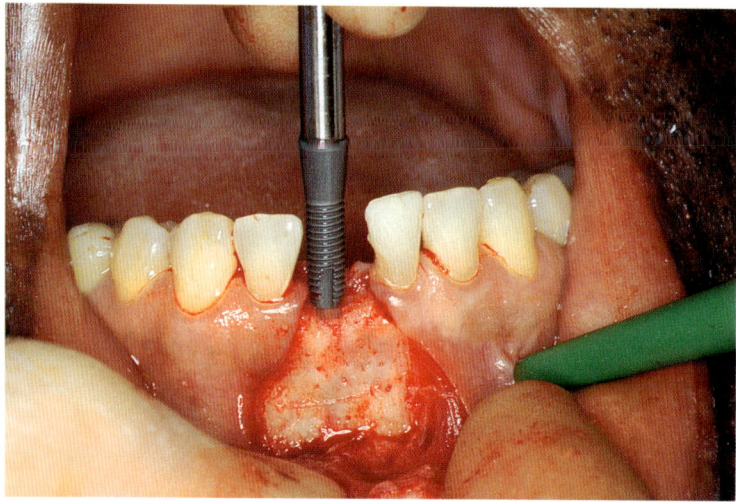

Fig 2-16 Other additional preparatory measures may be necessary to customise fixture sites to the design of an implant. The use of trephines is required for hollow implants and pictured here; a conical drill preparation is essential to receive the flared head of the Astra Single Tooth Implant.

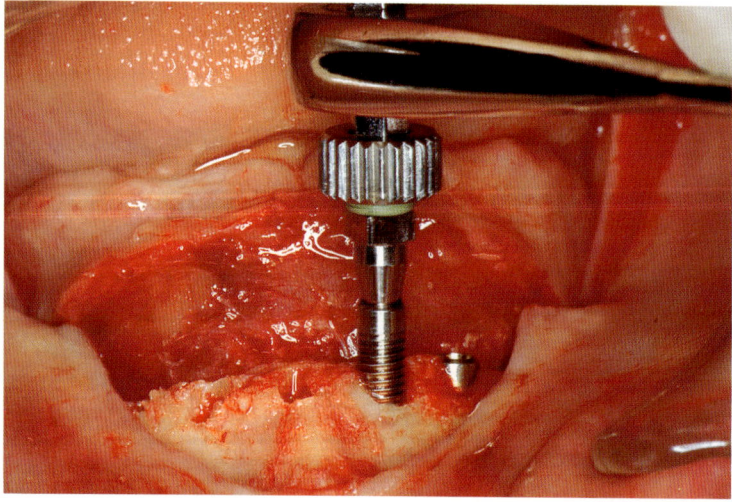

Fig 2-17 The insertion of any dental implant should be carried out in an atraumatic and controlled manner, either using a reducing handpiece running at 20 r.p.m. or as shown here, using a hand driven ratchet wrench. The need for irrigation is of course paramount.

implant has parallel sides. However for some implants there may now be one or two final preparatory steps in the surgery A term often mentioned when discussing implant surgery is countersinking, which refers to the need to crater the crestal bone (Fig 2-15), in order to receive the head of an implant which is, by design, wider than the implant body. When using the Astra single tooth implant, it is necessary to flare the coronal third of the implant preparation in order to receive the single tooth implant, which is flared to improve the aesthetic contour of the cervical margin of a single tooth restoration (Fig 2-16).

For screw type implants that are not self tapping, it is necessary as a final step to tap the bone prior to implant insertion. This tapping which cuts a thread into the bone, needs to be done at low speeds of 15-20 rpm. Likewise when inserting a self tapping implant, this should also be carried out at equivalent low speeds, which are controlled by using a hand ratchet instrument (Fig 2-17), or a high torque low speed handpiece to insert the implant. For press fit implants an instrument is usually provided to gently tap the implant into the bony socket.

It is now necessary to cover or occlude the implant surface which will interface with the transmucosal component (abutment), i.e. that component that relates the position of the implant into the oral cavity for bridge support. This is necessary to prevent bony overgrowth and subsequent seating problems.

Generally speaking there are two types of interface, internal or external. The external interface is usually associated with a flat topped implant that has a small hexagon, forming a butt joint with the cover screw and subsequent transmucosal components (Fig 2-18). The internal interface is usually of an hexagonal design as with the Screw Vent implant (Dentsply®/Implant Division, California, USA) or a conical or tapered design, as is presented by ITI implants (Institute Straumann AG, Waldenburg, Switzerland) and the Astra Tech Implant System (Astra Tech AB, Mölndal, Sweden) (Fig 2-19). Having secured these protective cover screws (Fig 2-20), the insertion procedure is complete.

Suturing

Prior to suturing, the surgical area is thoroughly irrigated and debrided. In suturing the wound, it is necessary to ensure that flaps are correctly repositioned, and that mattress sutures are employed to help evert the edges. The suture material of choice is somewhat subjective, but a 3/0 or 4/0 resorbable polyglactin suture (Vicryl®, Ethicon Ltd, Edinburgh, UK) is very suitable (Fig 2-21). The patient is now provided with an analgesic or non steroidal anti-inflammatory like Ibuprofen and asked to gently apply pressure to the wound with a damp gauze swab.

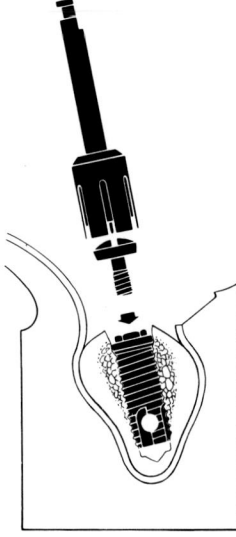

Fig 2-18 Insertion of the cover screw on a Brånemark implant, which demonstrates the external butt joint interface.

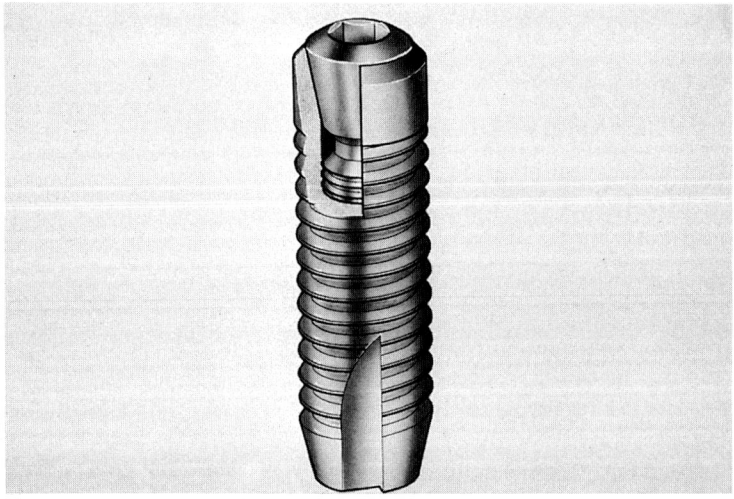

Fig 2-19 Both the Astra Tech Dental Implant and the ITI Im-implant advocate an internal conical or tapered interface which is occluded during healing by the insertion of a protective cover screw.

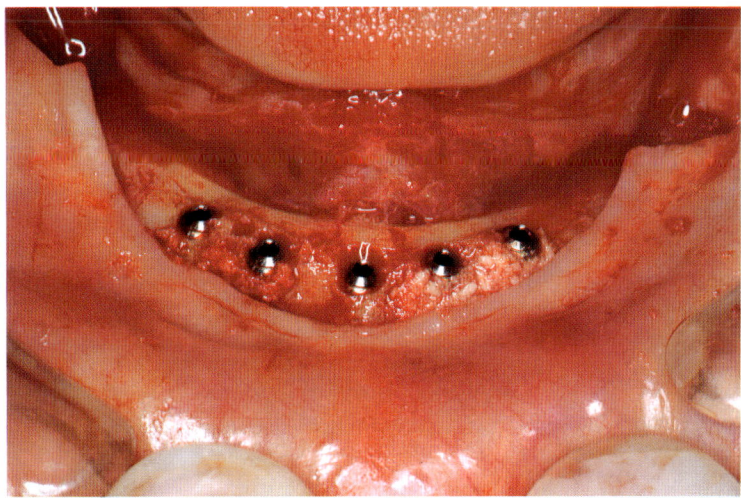

Fig 2-20 Five mandibular implants are shown, with their respective cover screws in situ. Note that the autogenous bone mush harvested earlier in the procedure has been used to patch up some of the crestal labial plate dehiscence that occurred during preparation.

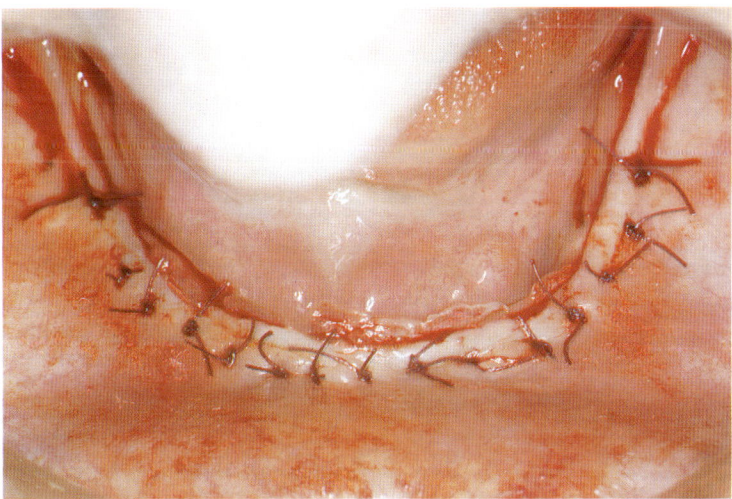

Fig 2-21 Tight and reliable suturing is essential. Multiple interrupted mattress sutures will ensure eversion of the edges and healing through primary intention. A weak suture will encourage exposure of the fixture heads through the overlying mucosa, which is contra-indicated in a two stage implant system.

Postoperative Management

This will include a prescription for antibiotics comparable to a 7 day course of Penicillin V, 250 mg QDS, analgesics when indicated, and a chlorhexidine mouthwash. The patient should be aware that there may be a need to leave the surgical site unencumbered by overlying prostheses, and as such it may be necessary not to wear dentures for a short period of time. Recommendations vary from two weeks to a few days, depending on whether the implants are proud of the marginal bone, or indeed left exposed in the mouth (see Chapter 3). However, all agree that it is necessary to thoroughly relieve that part of the prosthesis overlying the implants and in the case of a denture, this should be relined with a soft tissue conditioner like Viscogel® (De Trey Division, Dentsply Ltd., Surrey, England).

Though many general dental practitioners will refer patients for their implant surgery, they may well retain responsibility for overseeing the postoperative management of the patient. It is essential therefore to be aware of the exact position of the implants so that correct relief and relining can be effected.

Sutures are removed at one week and an assessment of soft tissue healing is noted. The patient should not now be neglected over the period of osseointegration but encouraged to attend clinic at least twice during this time to allow the dentist to oversee the healing of soft tissues and, in particular, to note the presence or absence of soft tissue perforation.

References

1   Adell, R., Lekholm, U., Rockler, B., Bråne-mark, P.-I. A 15-year study of osseointe-grated implants in the treatment of the edentulous jaw. Int J Oral Surg 1981; 10: 387-416.

2   Brånemark, P.-I., Breine, U., Adell, R., Hansson, B.O., Lindström, J., Olsson, Å. Intra-osseous anchorage of dental pros-theses. I. Experimental studies. Scand J Plast Reconstr Surg 1969; 3: 81-100.

3   Brånemark, P-I., Hansson, B.O., Adell, R., Breine, U., Lindström, J., Hallen, O., Öhman, A. Osseointegrated implants in the treat-ment of the edentulous jaw. Experience from a 10-year period. Scand J Plast Reconstr Surg 1977; 11: Suppl 16.

4   Albrektsson, T., Brånemark, P.-I., Hansson, H.A., Lindström, J. Osseointegrated titanium implants. Acta Orthop Scand 1981; 52: 155-170.

5   Cranin, N.A., Rabkin, M.F., Garfinkel, L. A statistical evaluation of 952 endosteal im-plants in humans. J Am Dent Assoc 1977; 94: 315-320.

6   Zarb, G.A., Smith, D.C., Levant, H.C., Graham, B.S., Zing, G.W. The effects of cemented and uncemented endosseous im-plants. J Prosthet Dont 1979; 42: 202-210.

7   Eriksson, R.A. Heat induced bone tissue injury. An in vivo investigation of heat tolerance of bone tissue and temperature rise in the drilling of cortical bone. Thesis, University of Göteborg 1984.

8   Eriksson, R.A., Albrektsson, T. Temperature threshold levels for heat-induced bone tissue injury: A vital microscopic study in the rabbit. J Prosthet Dent 1983; 50: 101-107.

9   Eriksson, R.A., Albrektsson, T. The effect of heat on bone regeneration. J Oral Maxil-lofac Surg 1984; 42: 705-711.

10 Eriksson, R.A., Adell, R. Temperatures during drilling for the placement of implants using the osseointegration technique. J Oral Maxillofac Surg 1986; 44: 4-7.

11 Watanabe, F., Tawada, Y., Komatsu, S., Hata, Y. Heat distribution in bone during preparation of implant sites: Heat analysis by real-time thermography. Int J Oral Maxil-lofac Implants 1992; 7: 212-219.

12 Haider, R., Watzek, G., Plenk, H. Effects of drill cooling and bone structure on IMZ implant fixation. Int J Oral Maxillofac Im-plants 1993; 8: 83-91.

3 Location and Exposure of Implants

Submerged or Transmucosal

As a rule, the majority of implant manufacturers support the concept that implants should be submerged below the mucosa during the healing or osseointegration phase and that this is an essential requirement for predictable implant success.[1-4]

The soft tissues are tightly sutured over the implants, thus isolating them from the intra-oral microbial environment and protecting them from the loading of a temporary overlying prosthesis.

Consequently, it is necessary to locate these implants, identifying their position with a probe (Fig 3-1), and perhaps, utilising the original surgical template to expose them through the overlying soft tissues, prior to prosthodontic procedures. It would therefore seem correct to consider this a second surgical procedure, but with the advent of the temporary healing abutment (transmucosal post), any surgery required is often minimal and ensures that the selection of the final abutment can be left to the prosthodontist. It must also be recognised that the ITI Implant System today advocates a single stage or transmucosal approach[5-7] which leaves implants exposed from the day of insertion.

This has important ramifications for the team approach, removing the burden of abutment selection from the surgeon, who simply places a standard temporary healing abutment with minimal trauma to the patient. This then leaves the critical decision making to the prosthodontist, who will be more aware of the requirements of the final abutments.

At this stage it is now possible to ascertain the surgical success of implant osseointegration. The criteria used to denote implant success are for the greater part subjective. In 1986 Albrektsson et al., proposed an update[8] of minimal criteria previously proposed,[9] and which are still used today as the guide for assessing the success of new implant systems. These criteria are reproduced in Table 3-1. However it should be noted that these criteria are for the most part, time dependent, leaving little scope for assessing implant success at exposure.

Table 3-1   Criteria for Implant Success

Albrektsson, Zarb, Worthington and Eriksson, 1986

1   That an individual, unattached implant is immobile when tested clinically.
2   That a radiograph does not demonstrate any evidence of peri-implant radiolucency.
3   That vertical bone loss be less than 0.2mm annually following the implant's first year of service.
4   That individual implant performance be characterised by an absence of persistent and/or irreversible signs and symptoms such as pain, infections, neuropathies, paraesthesia, or violation of the mandibular canal.
5   That, in the context of the above, a successful rate of 85% at the end of a five-year observation period and 80% at the end of a ten-year period be a minimum criterion for success.

Some effort has been made in using the Periotest® (Siemens AG, Bensheim, Germany) to provide an objective, measurable, clinical diagnosis of bone-implant apposition[10] for early assessment, but for the majority, a reliance on radiographic evaluation, the absence of mobility, pain and/or infection and the presence of a metallic ringing tone on implant percussion, remain the only sources for determining implant success.

Whether using the Periotest® or simply the handle of a dental mirror for percussion, the result will be influenced by the implant/abutment interface. If not accurately apposed, as a result of inaccurate seating, or tissue trapping, this will give either a false positive or a dull percussion note. Reflecting on the criteria above, it is clear that an indication of early success, should only be considered in the context of long term functional success and is therefore only the first of many opportunities that should be taken to measure or assess implant viability.

The healing abutment (Fig 3-2) which allows for a period of soft tissue maturation, is placed through a punch or slit incision (Fig 3-3) to locate the implant exposed below (Fig 3-4). Locating abutments correctly on those implants with a hex top external interface can be time consuming and protocol recommends that all abutments, particularly the final abutments, are checked for correct seating by means of an intra-oral radiograph. With the internal conical interface all abutments are self guiding and it is not possible for the abutment to be seated incorrectly.

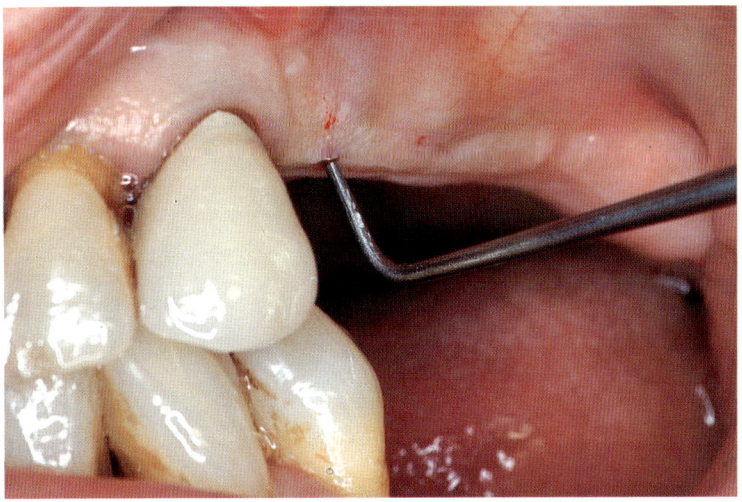

Fig 3-1 Implants are identified first on a radiograph and then a probe is used to locate the domed cover screw below. Reuse of the surgical stent might help in their location.

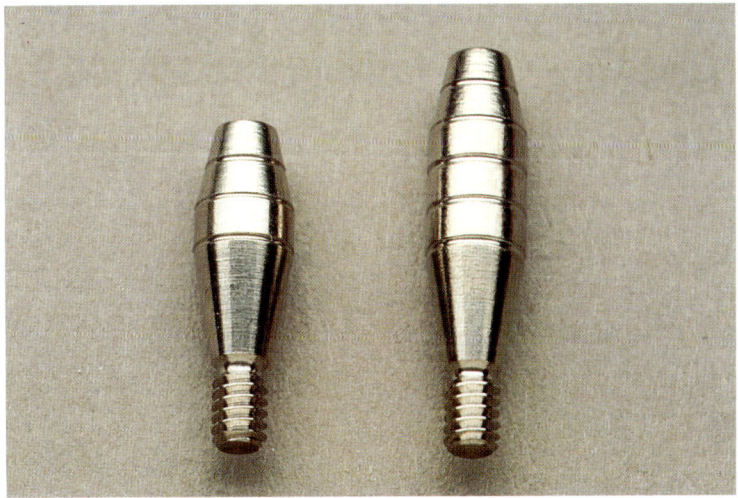

Fig 3-2 Healing abutments are widely used as temporary trans-mucosal components, allowing peri-implant soft tissues to mature, prior to final abutment seating. The presence of grooves, which act as *in situ* soft tissue depth markers, enables the clinician to accurately select the correct length of final abutment.

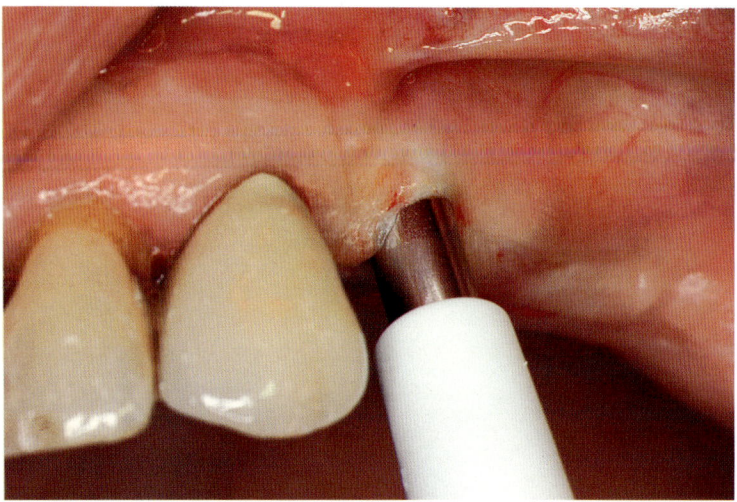

Fig 3-3 Cover screws are exposed through a slit or punch incision, avoiding the need to strip periosteum. The punch is not indicated where only a narrow band of keratinised tissue exists.

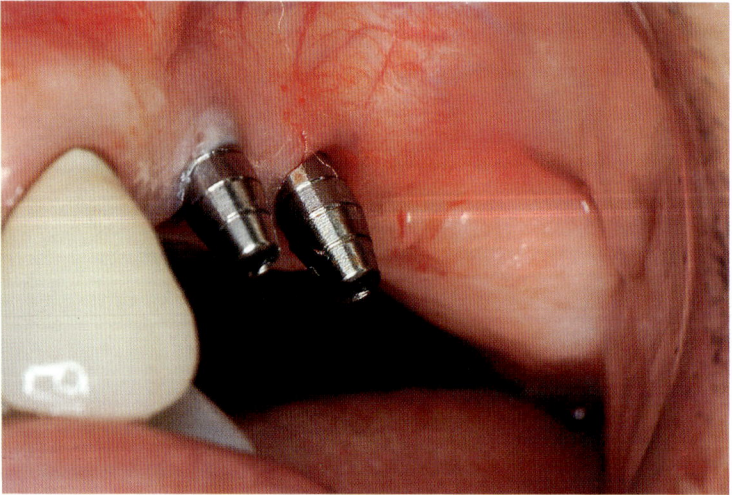

Fig 3-4 Healing abutments are inserted directly to engage the internal conical interface. All three depth grooves are clearly visible, which would indicate that the shortest Uni-abutments™ will be selected.

It is advisable to irrigate the interface and flush out any debris with chlorhexidine prior to seating the healing abutments. The reader is directed to manufacturer recommendations with respect to the handling and seating of abutments, as this will vary between systems.

The advantage of a submerged implant is that the marginal metal collar of the implant is placed well below the mucosal margin. In recognition of the much higher aesthetic standards which are demanded today, even the transmucosal implants are pseudo-submerged, with an extension healing cap that acts in a similar manner to the healing abutment.

Healing abutments are usually left in situ for approximately two weeks post insertion, during which time soft tissues mature to form a tight cuff around the abutment. This has been shown to adhere to the surface via hemidesmosonal attachments, with an organised inner implant epithelium of non-keratinised, flattened squamous cells covering a collagenous stroma.[11] Fibres within the stroma generally run either parallel to the abutment surface or as a circular network, as recently shown around the transmucosal variety.[12]

On removing the healing abutments, or extended healing caps, a firm soft tissue cuff should demonstrate tone, that is it should not collapse and there should be an absence of bleeding (Fig 3-5). No local anaesthetic is generally required on removing these temporary transmucosal components.

It is now possible to measure soft tissue thickness using a periodontal probe or a purpose designed soft tissue depth gauge (Fig 3-6) giving direct readings for the final abutment length. In figure 3-2 the healing abutment is seen to be graded with grooves that correspond to the available final abutment lengths, thus acting directly as an in situ soft tissue depth gauge.

The selection of final abutments will depend on:

1 Technical considerations (Fixed bridge or overdenture treatment)
2 Functional considerations (Occlusion, guidance and parafunction)
3 Aesthetic considerations (Implant position and patient perception)
4 Hygiene considerations (Access and manual dexterity)

Inter-occlusal space, access for instrumentation, implant position and inclination, may all further influence the decision of final abutment selection.

The variety of abutment designs even outweighs the plethora of implants, potentially making life for the novice even more confusing. It is not the intention of this chapter to offer an inventory for different designs. Only standard abutments will be described, drawing particular attention to the difference between one and two piece abutment designs. For those implants that present an

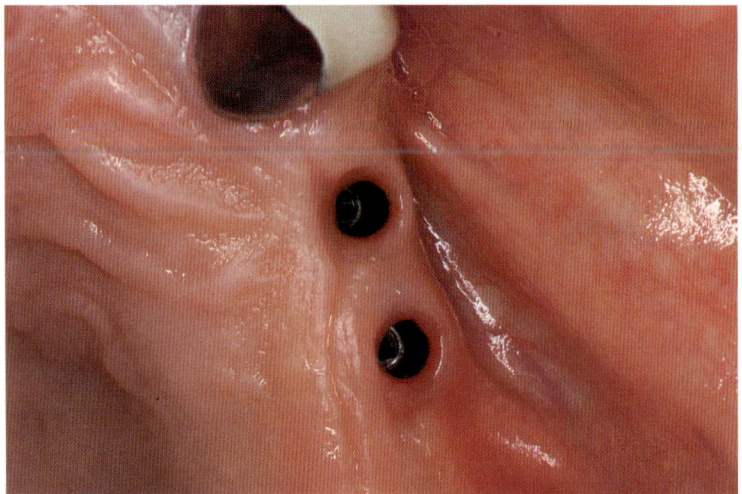

Fig 3-5 After approximately two weeks of soft tissue maturation, healing abutments are removed to reveal a healthy peri-implant cuff, that should demonstrate tone and be absent of frank bleeding.

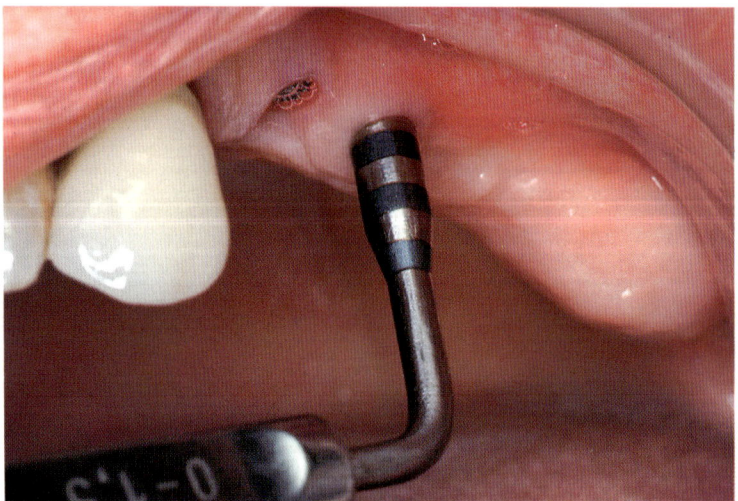

Fig 3-6 If necessary soft tissue thickness can be assessed using a soft tissue depth gauge, which is indicated when healing abutments are not used, or for those systems where graded healing abutments are not available.

hexagonal anti-rotation device on top of the fixture, it is necessary for the abutment to be constructed in two pieces (Fig 3-7). The first piece is the transmucosal collar which engages the hexagonal part of the fixture head. The second piece, the abutment screw, passes through the middle of the collar screwing into the fixture, thus uniting the fixture and abutment collar with a butt joint interface.

For those implants with an internal conical interface, abutments are designed as one piece units (Fig 3-8) that screw directly into the fixture. Though no claims are offered for anti-rotation, the concept of a Conical Seal Design™ (Astra Tech AB, Mölndal, Sweden) has been shown to impart superior strength and support at the implant abutment interface.[13]

For single tooth restorations it is essential to have an anti-rotation feature between the fixture and abutment. The next chaper will deal with this specific restoration in greater detail.

For the system being described in this text, there are two types of standard, Uni-Abutment™, with a 20° or 45° tapered top (Fig 3-9). These permanent abutments are selected for fixed bridgework or overdenture treatment respectively. The 45° abutment is also useful for those situations where inter-occlusal space precludes the use of the 20° abutment for fixed bridgework; conversely the 20° abutment can be used for bar type overdenture attachments to provide additional support against lateral loads.

The details of abutment selection for individual prostheses will be discussed in subsequent chapters. However the insertion of abutments is considered below.

Having removed the healing abutment and measured soft tissue depth, the relevant final abutment is selected and mounted on the abutment adapter (Fig 3-10). Care should be taken not to damage the delicate threading of the bridge screw hole. The conical interface is flushed with chlorhexidine and the permanent abutment is secured either with light finger pressure or using a torque controller as dictated by manufacturer recommendations, to ensure complete seating (Fig 3-11). If a hex top implant is being utilised it is essential to take an intra-oral radiograph to confirm accurate seating of the abutment. With the final abutments in place, subsequent restorative procedures can begin.

Between visits, small plastic protective caps can be secured to the abutments to prevent food impaction into the bridge screw holes and to avoid any damage.

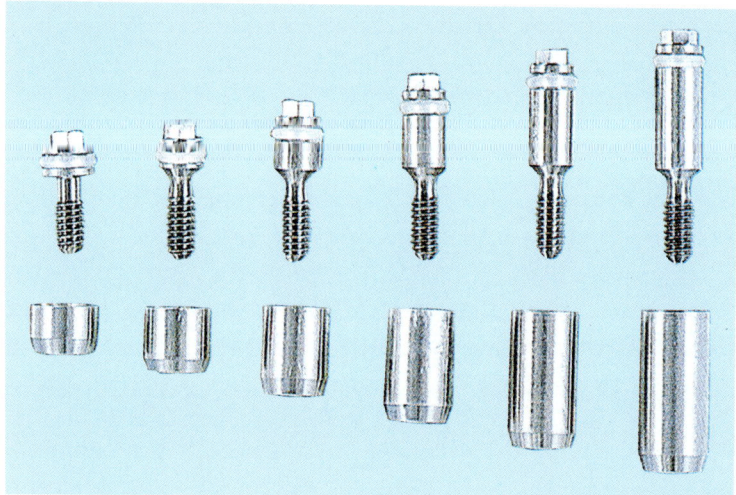

Fig 3-7 Two piece abutments comprise a hollow cylinder of various lengths with a central abutment screw that secures the cylinder to the implant. In the system shown (Brånemark) a plastic ring is used to seal the communicating channel between intra-oral and submucosal environments.

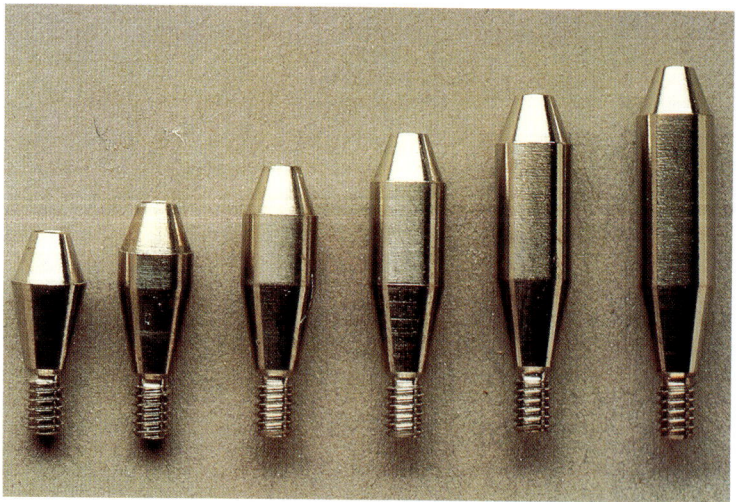

Fig 3-8 One piece abutments screw directly in to the fixture and are solid components. There is no internal communication between intra-oral and submucosal environments.

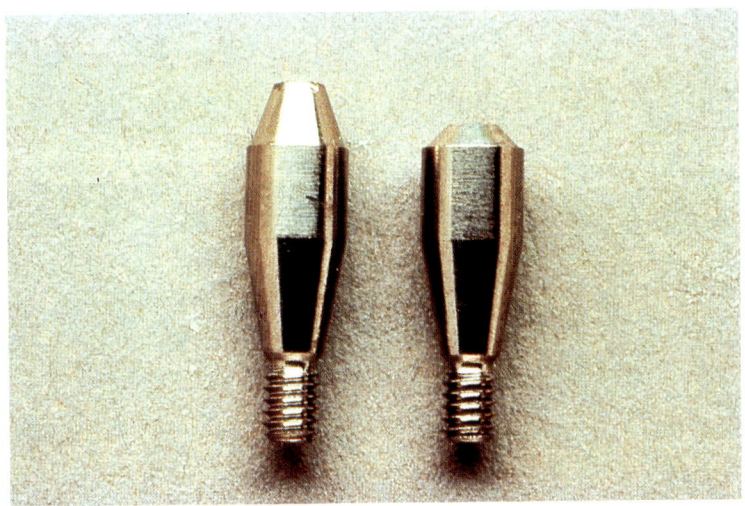

Fig 3-9 The Astra abutment is presented with the option of a 20° tapered top, or a 45° tapered top. These are used for fixed bridge and/or overdenture treatment respectively.

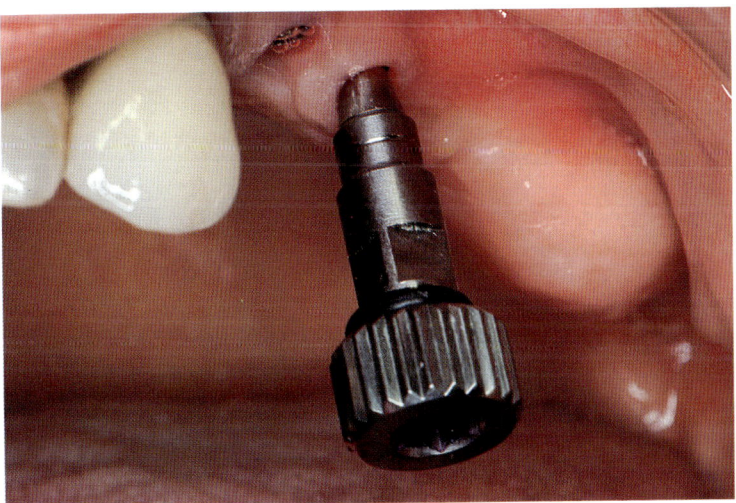

Fig 3-10 Permanent Uni-abutments™ are located using an abutment adapter. Due to the precise fit and guidance of the internal Conical Seal Design™, only light finger pressure is required for accurate seating. In this case no radiographs are required to confirm correct abutment sealing.

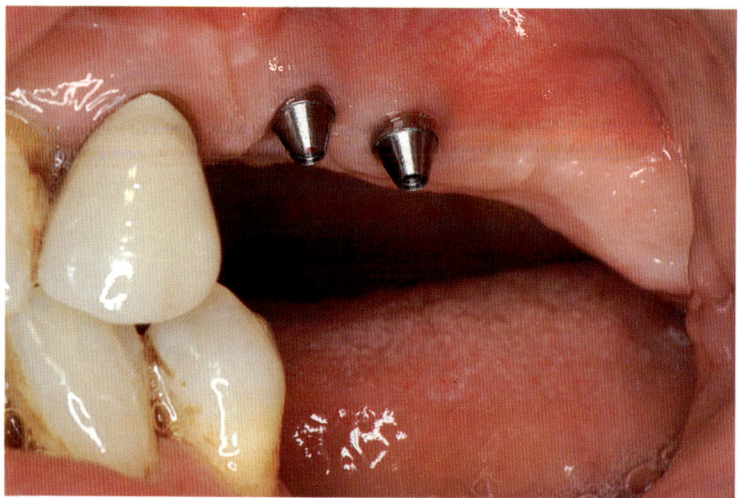

Fig 3-11 Final abutments are shown above *in situ*. It is now possible for the prosthodontist to take impressions and embark on the prosthetic rehabilitation (See chapter 5).

References

1 Adell, R., Lekholm, U., Rockler, B., Bråne-mark, P.-I. A 15-year study of osseointe-grated implants in the treatment of the edentulous jaw. Int J Oral Surg 1981; 10: 387-416.

2 Arvidson, K., Bystedt, H., Frykholm, A., von Konow, L., Lothigius, E. A 3-year clinical study of Astra dental implants in the treat-ment of edentulous mandibles. Int J Oral Maxillofac Implants 1992; 7: 321-329.

3 Niznick, G.A. The Core-Vent implant system. J Oral Implantol 1982; 10: 379-418.

4 Kirsch, A., Ackerman, K.L. The IMZ osseo-integrated implant system. Dent Clin North Am 1989; 33: 733-761.

5 Buser, D.A., Schroeder, A., Sutter, F., Lang, N.P. The new concept of ITI hollow-cylinder and hollow-screw implants: Part 2. Clinical aspects, indications, and early clinical results. Int J Oral Maxillofac Implants 1988; 3: 173-181.

6 Buser, D.A., Weber, H.P., Brägger, U., Bal-siger, C. Tissue integration of one-stage ITI implants: 3-year results of a longitudinal study with hollow-cylinder and hollow-screw implants. Int J Oral Maxillofac Implants 1991; 6: 405-412.

7 Jennings, K.J., Critchlow, H.A., Lilly, P., Broad, M.T. The clinical use of ITI trans-mucosal implants. Brit Dent J 1992; 173: 67-71.

8 Albrektsson, T., Zarb, G.A., Worthington, P., Eriksson, A.R. The long-term efficacy of currently used dental implants: A review and proposed criteria for success. Int J Oral Maxillofac Implants 1986; 1: 11-25.

9 Schnitman, P.A., Shulman, L.B. Recom-mendations of the consensus development conference on dental implants. J Am Dent Assoc 1979; 98: 373-377.

10 Teerlinck, J., Quirynen, M., Darius, P., van Steenberghe, D. Periotest®: An objective clinical diagnosis of bone apposition toward implants. J Oral Maxillofac Implants 1991; 6: 55-61.

11 Arvidson, K. Bystedt, H., Ericsson, I. Histo-metric and ultrastructural studies of tissues surrounding Astra dental implants in dogs. Int J Oral Maxillofac Implants 1990; 5: 127-134.

12 Ruggeri, A., Franchi, M., Marini, N., Trisi, P., Piattelli, A. Supracrestal circular col-lagen fiber network around nonsubmerged titanium implants. Clin Oral Impl Res 1992; 3: 169-175.

13 A comparative study of the mechanical strength of the Astra implant fixture-abut-ment interface versus the Brånemark im-plant fixture-abutment interface. Personal communication, Swedish National Research and Testing Institute, Borås, Sweden.

4 Single Tooth Replacement (STR)

Whilst STR is perhaps the most exciting advance in implant technology, with the general practitioner expressing a great deal of interest in this particular area, it is nonetheless a most demanding and difficult restoration.

The unique requirements of STR have been considered by the experts to be complex, though it is recognised that STR may well become the most sought after treatment referred by the general practitioner. It therefore rightly takes precedent in this prosthodontic section.

Prior to tackling STR it is necessary to have an appreciation of the causes of tooth loss or absence.[1] It is useful to consider the surgical sieve and to determine if tooth loss is developmental or acquired and furthermore whether the acquired condition is the result of trauma, infection, or pathology. As a rule it is worth remembering that *the ideal restoration should not be compromised by the cause of tooth loss; and should itself not compromise general dental health.*

Requirements for STR have been listed in Table 4.1 and for con-venience are split into surgical and prosthodontic sections.

The loss of an anterior single tooth can have a profound effect on the appearance of an individual (Fig 4-1), often resulting in social embarrassment. Concerted efforts have recently been made in the implant field to accommodate STR within the remit of implant therapy and already a number of articles have been published discussing this treatment concept.[2-7]

An essential technical requirement has been the construction of an abutment that provides dual anti-rotation, not only between fixture and abutment (already available for the hex top implants) but also between the abutment and the crown, which being unsplinted would be subject to loosening under torquing forces.

Furthermore it was recognised that the average implant width would not lend itself to supporting a crown with an aesthetic optimal profile as it emerged through the soft tissues. New abutment designs were required, that would incorporate dual anti-rotation features and help improve the crown emergence profile.

Table 4-1   Local Indications and Requirements for Use of a Single Tooth Implant

Surgical	Prosthodontic
Absence of local pathology or infection	Available saddle width (with respect to component specifications)
Adequate bone volume	Available interocclusal space
Suitable socket status or ridge morphology	Occlusal factors, ie Anterior/canine guidance, group function and contact scheme
Acceptable bone quality	Absence of parafunction
Healthy soft tissue status	Crown: implant ratio = 1:2
Absence of vital structures in the surgical field	Minimally restored adjacent teeth

A number of publications have presented various options available for use with a variety of hex top implant designs.[8-11]

The system demonstrated in this book so far, has presented an internal conical design that does not incorporate any anti-rotational mechanism. It was therefore necessary for the manufacturers to design a single tooth system which should incorporate dual anti-rotation features and an improved emergence profile to accommodate the needs of STR. This chapter will introduce the concept of STR using this system.

Having determined that an implant is the optimum treatment of choice (according to those guidelines set out in chapter 1) and that it will promote and not compromise general dental health (Fig 4-2), the basic surgical protocol is unchanged, with incision, flap elevation (Fig 4-3) and bone preparation (Fig 4-4) following similar lines to those described in chapter 2.

Additional care is required in the handling of soft tissues to ensure that at least 1 mm of interdental tissue is left intact (Fig 4-3). This is necessary in order to maintain a functional and aesthetic interdental papilla which will otherwise recede if it is stripped along with the mucoperiosteal flap. Furthermore it is also necessary to adapt the bone site to the design of the fixture. In this case the use of a conical drill (Fig 4-5) flares the coronal aspect of the bony site (Fig 4-6) to meet the geometry of the single tooth fixture (See Fig 2-16).

The surface texture of this single tooth implant is roughened by a cleaning process that blasts titanium dioxide particles at the implant (TiOblast™) thus roughening the surface available for osseointegration by a pitting of the titanium. This has been shown to result in an

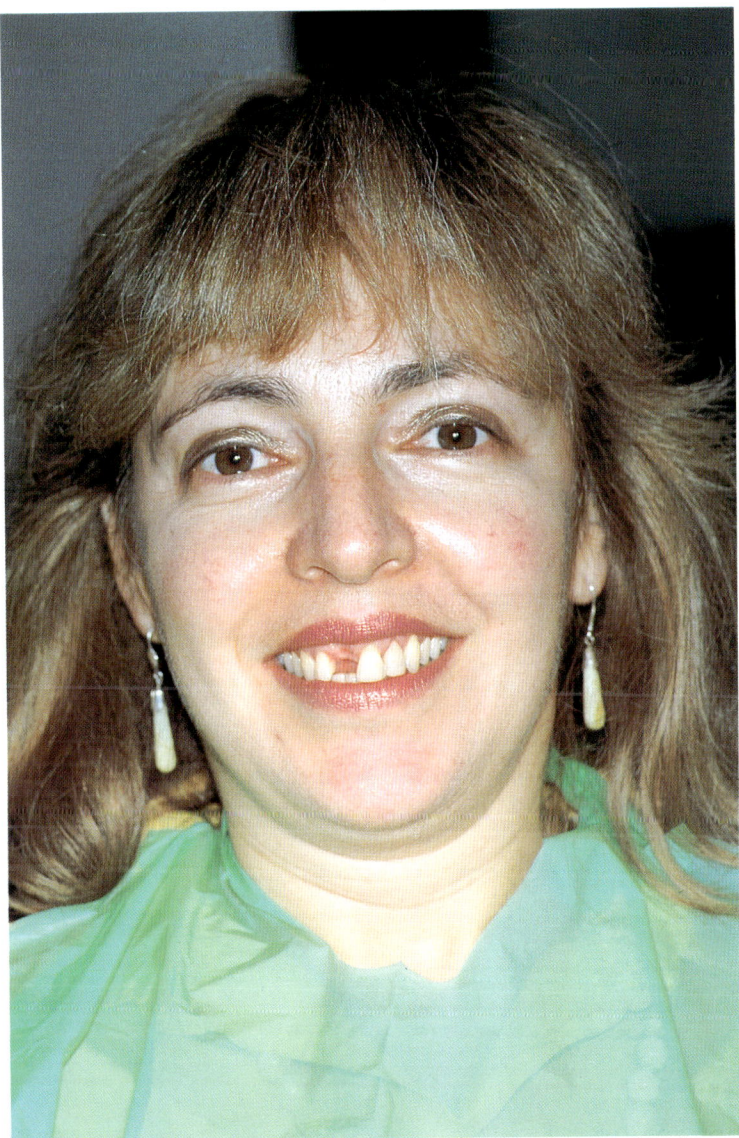

Fig 4-1 Loss or absence of a tooth can be emotionally upsetting and socially embarrassing as well as compromising function and the ideal dental state. A glance at the completed restoration (Fig 4-23, p78) will show the difference that can be made.

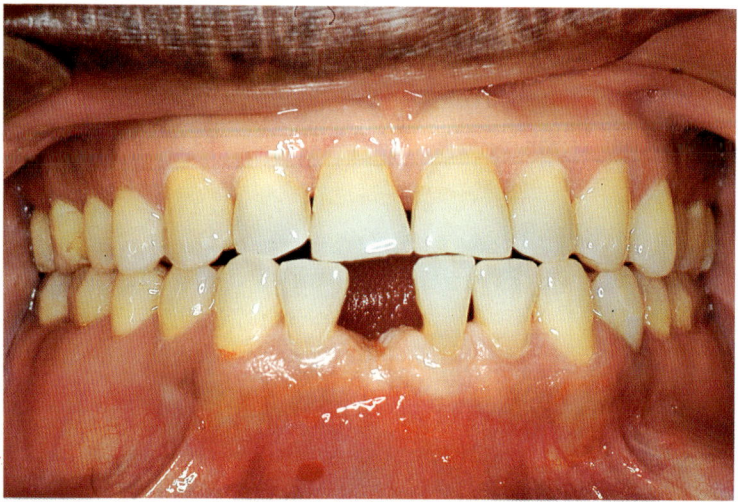

Fig 4-2 An ideal case for implant replacement. All adjacent tissues demonstrate health and vitality and the provision of an implant would prove more conservative than other more conventional restorations.

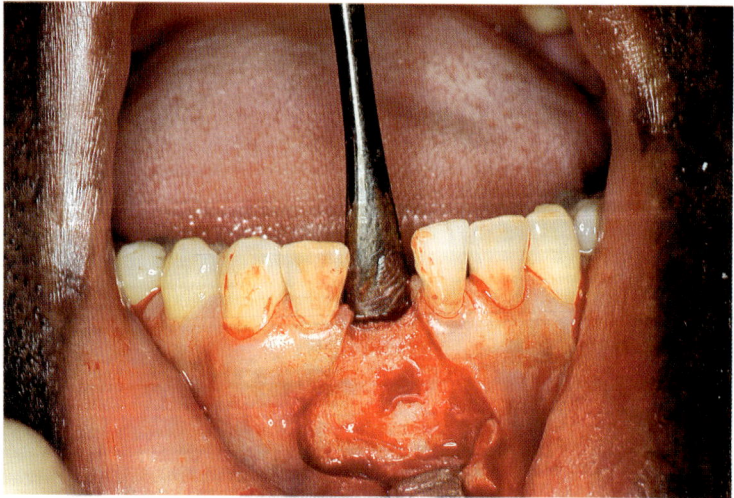

Fig 4-3 For single tooth replacement, the incision line and mucoperiosteal flap should leave a 1 mm margin of sound interdental tissue unstripped from the underlying bone. This will ensure the maintenance of aesthetically pleasing papillae, enhancing the contour and shade of the porcelain restoration.

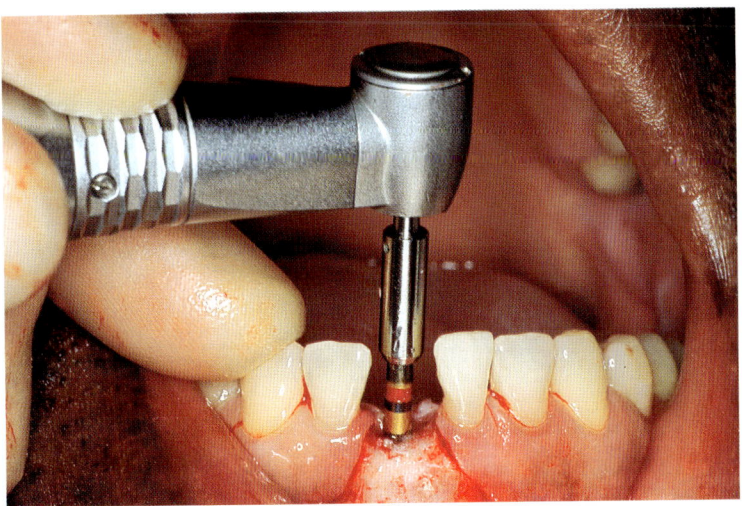

Fig 4-4 Bone preparation is carried out in the manner described in chapter 2. The need for a drill extension connector is often indicated when placing an implant between adjacent natural teeth.

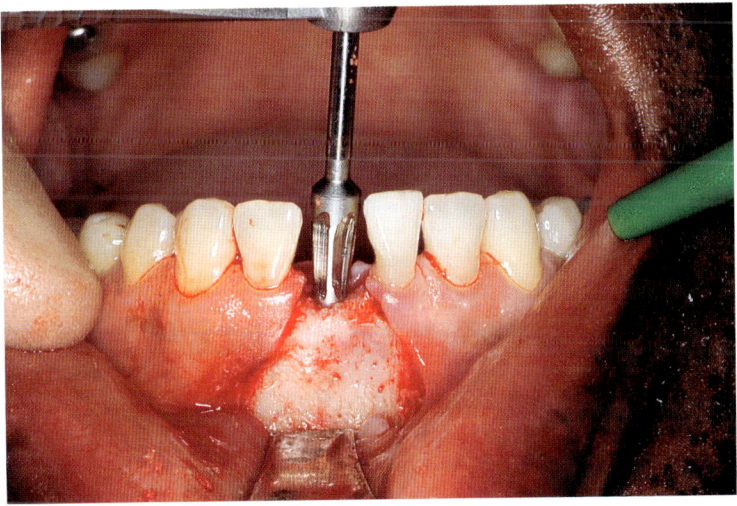

Fig 4-5 The need to customise bone preparation, according to implant design, is highlighted here by the use of a conical drill for the flared Astra single tooth implant.

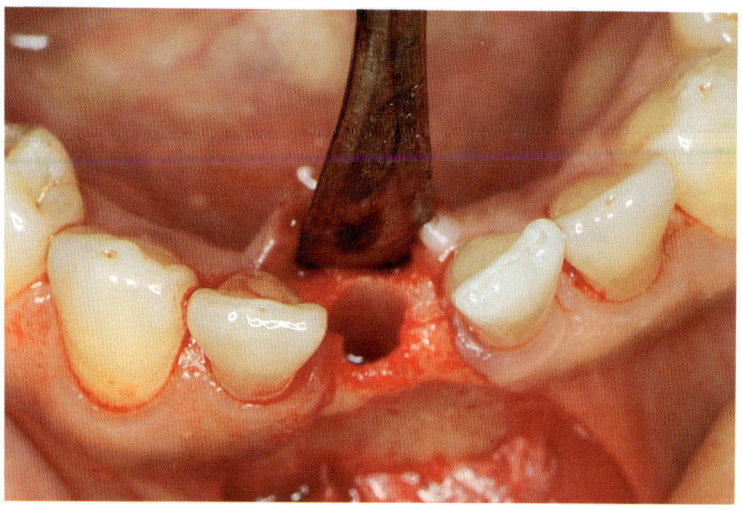

Fig 4-6 Ideally the host bone site should comfortably accommodate the preparation, without resulting in fenestrations or perforations. The use of accurate ridge mapping techniques will encourage predictable results.

increased resistance to torquing forces[12] and may have an impact on the rate and degree of osseointegration.[13] Similar results have been claimed for titanium plasma spray and hydroxyapatite coatings.[14-17] Additionally *Microthreads*™ characterise the flared coronal part (Fig 4-7), ensuring that osseointegration is achieved even at the most coronal aspect of the fixture.

Healing periods follow standard protocol, as does the exposure of the implant through a slit or punch incision (Fig 4-8). Having ascertained mucosal thickness (Fig 4-9), it is then possible to insert the single tooth abutment (Fig 4-10), securing it to the fixture with a central abutment screw. The single tooth abutment is characterised by an internal hex at the base of the conical interface, with an external *Octagonal Star Design*™ that provides anti-rotation between crown and abutment (Fig 4-11). The concave surfaces of the octagon also act as cement venting reservoirs, preventing excess cement from interfering with crown seating (Fig 4-12).

Impression techniques are made simple by utilising a prefabricated plastic impression coping which is similar for a number of systems (Fig 4-13). The ideal impression material of choice is Impregum® (ESPE, Oberbay, W. Germany) being a relatively mobile material on inser-

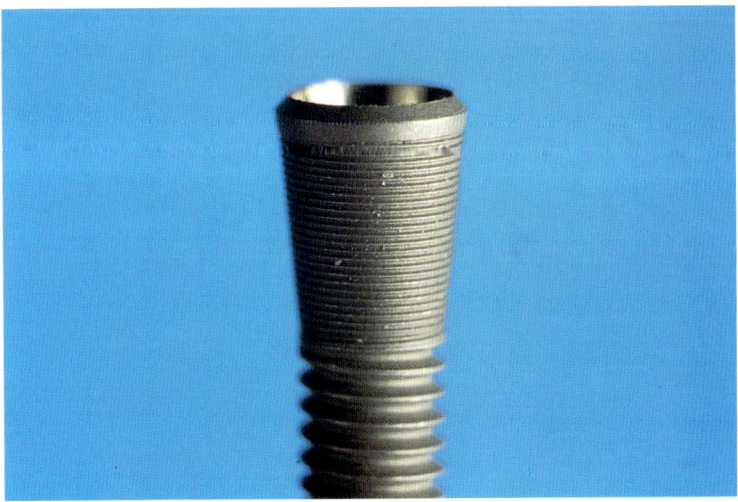

Fig 4-7 The Astra single tooth implant is characterised by a TiOblast™ surface with coronal Microthreading™ which optimises interfacial surface area and encourages predictable osseointegration.

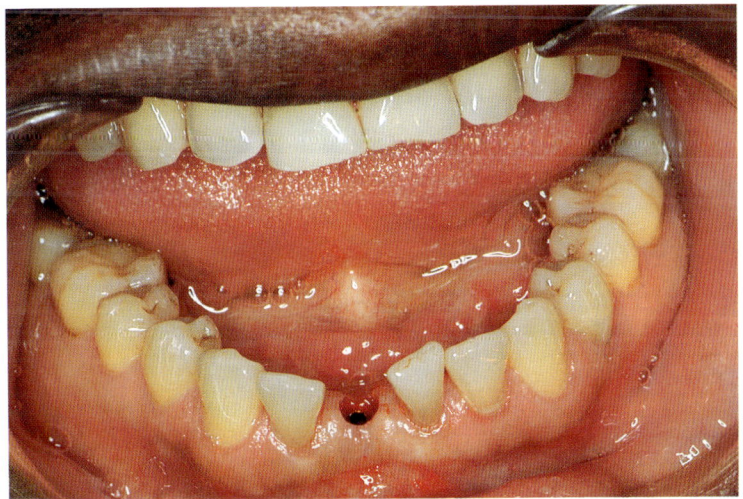

Fig 4-8 The underlying cover screw is exposed through a slit or punch incision.

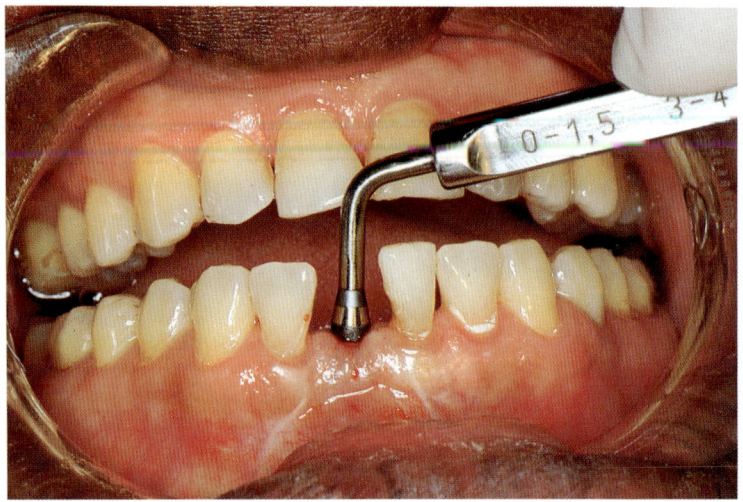

Fig 4-9 Soft tissue thickness is measured with a depth gauge that locates directly into the fixture. Readings correspond with available abutment lengths.

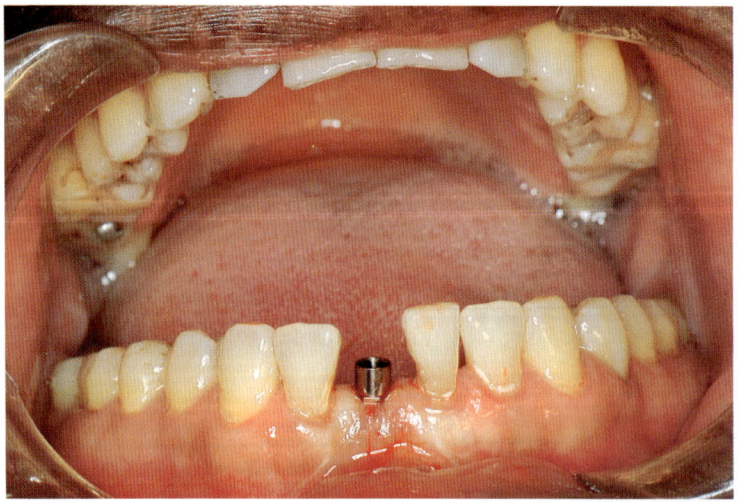

Fig 4-10 The abutment locates the internal hexagon of the fixture and is secured to it by means of an abutment screw, which passes through the centre of the hollow abutment.

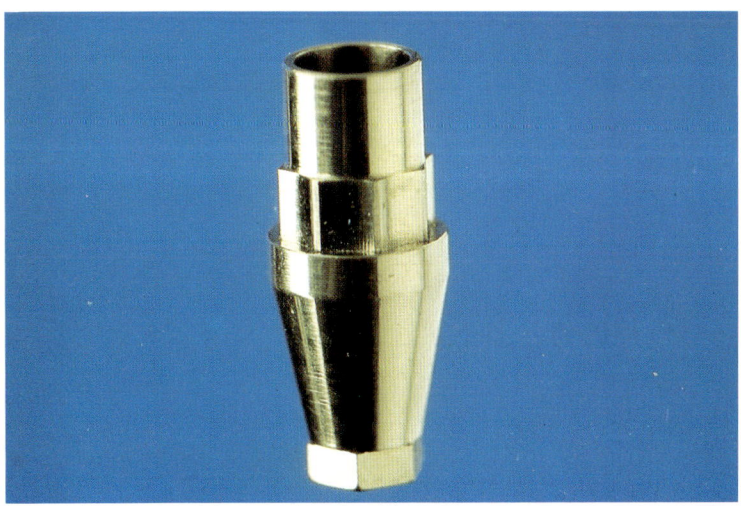

Fig 4-11 The Astra single tooth abutment is characterised by a locating hex at the base of the conical interface; an external Octagonal Star Design™ for abutment/crown anti-rotation; and a cylindrical body for support of the restoration.

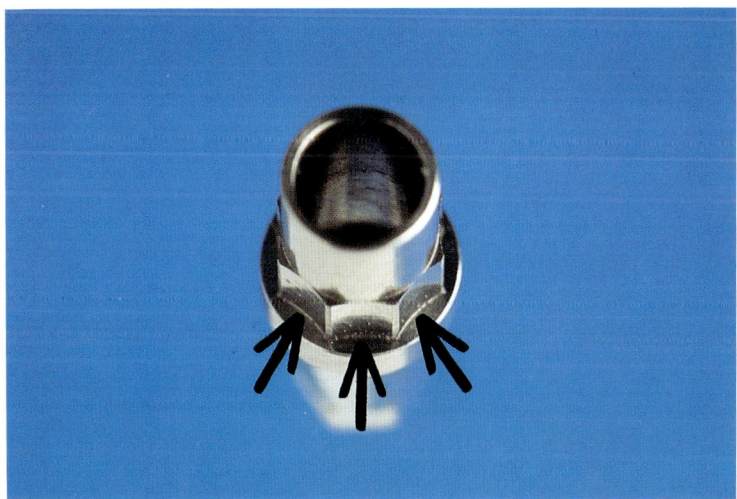

Fig 4-12 The Octagonal Star Design™ incorporates concavities that act as venting reservoirs, to allow the free flow and accommodation of excess cement, thus preventing mis-seating of the crown due to hydrostatic pressure caused by excess cement in a confined space.

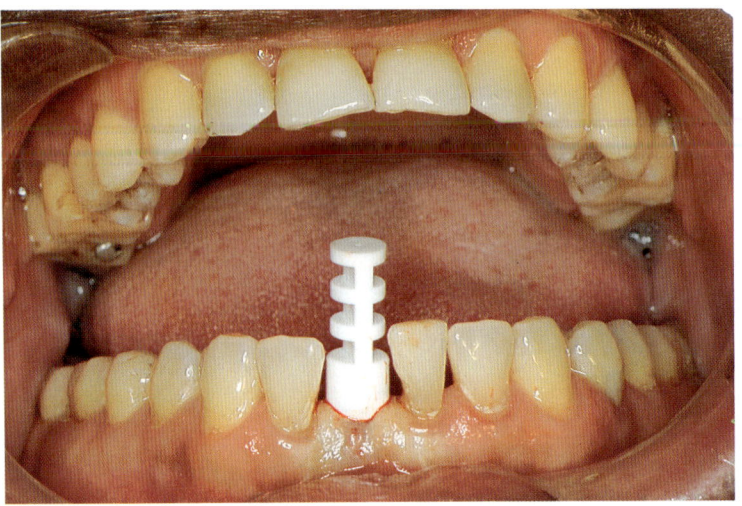

Fig 4-13 Plastic friction fit copings are secured to the abutment for the impression. Retention tags ensure that the coping is withdrawn with the impression.

tion, yet withdrawable whilst being rigid at final set.

It is essential that the impression coping is accurately seated on the abutment. On inspection of the impression (Fig 4-14), any material apparent on the inside of the coping is indicative of inaccurate seating and obligates a retake of the impression. The use of a stock tray is acceptable for single implant impressions; however for multiple implant impressions it may be preferable to arrange for a customised tray to be fabricated.

The patient will require temporisation while the impression is sent to the laboratory for casting and crown fabrication. In the system demon-strated an impression coping can be cut to size and cold cured acrylic bonded to it for aesthetics (Fig 4-15). Though some systems have historically advocated the manufacture of implant borne prostheses on stone die replicas of the abutments,[18] the majority of implant manufacturers today recommend the use of laboratory abutment replicas (or analogues), which are inexpensive steel dummies that are incorporated into the master cast (Fig 4-16). In keeping with the concept of accuracy, most single tooth systems provide a prefabricated gold alloy cylinder to act as the fitting surface of the crown. Alternatively the Bråne-mark system also provides a pre-

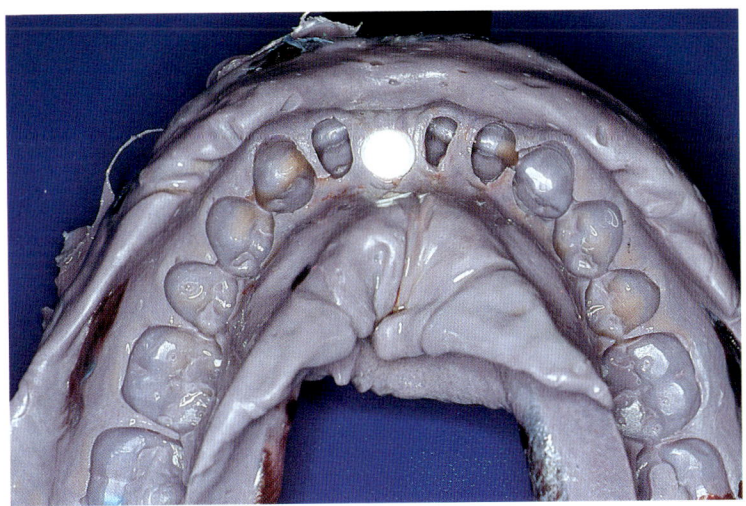

Fig 4-14 Impregum® (ESPE, Oberbay, W. Germany) impression material with coping *in situ*. Any material on the fitting surface of the coping would denote inaccurate seating, requiring the impression to be retaken.

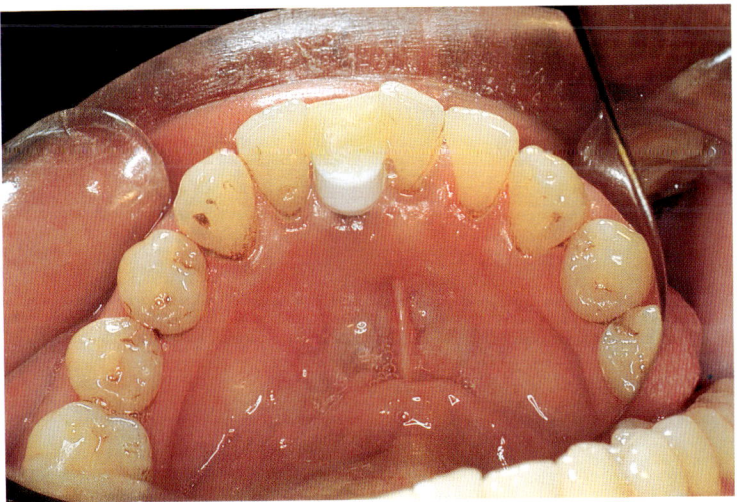

Fig 4-15 A separate coping can be cut down and used for temporisation, between visits. Cold cured acrylic can be bonded to the coping to restore tooth form.

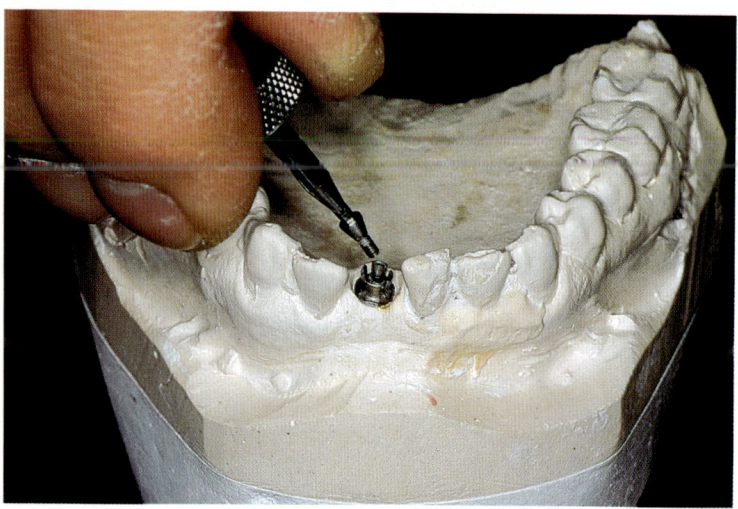

Fig 4-16 Steel or brass laboratory replicas are secured in to the coping, prior to casting. The set master cast will then incorporate an accurate analogue, on which the final restoration can be fabricated. In this case a securing screw will help to keep the casting cylinder firmly on the replica.

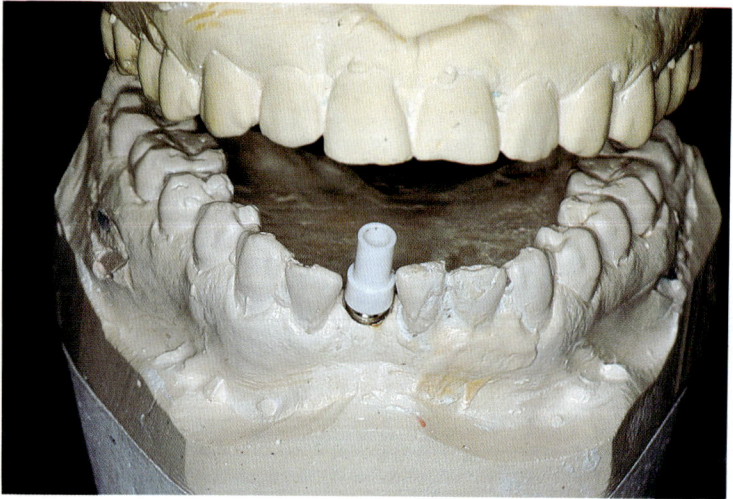

Fig 4-17 In order to achieve an accurate fit, the metalwork for the crown is cast around a prefabricated gold alloy cylinder which locates on to the abutment replica. The press fit plastic sheath is helpful during the waxing procedure.

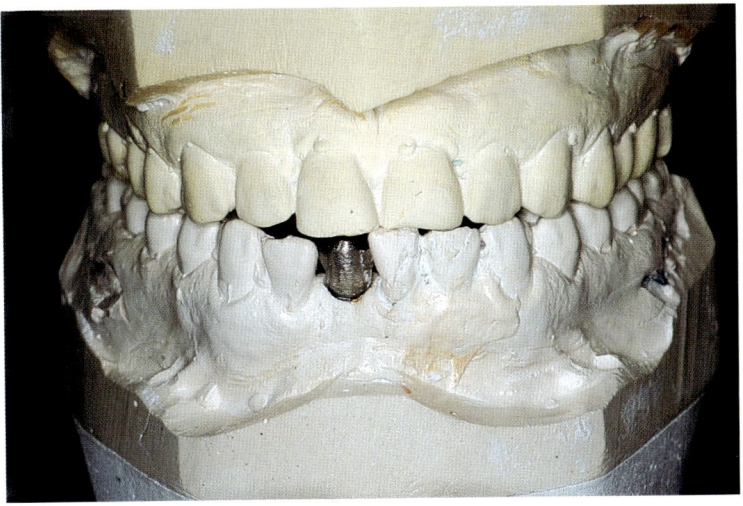

Fig 4-18 Metalwork can be cast in precious or semi precious bonding alloys. However different systems produce cylinders in different alloys and it is therefore necessary to confirm with the manufacturer, which casting metals are suitable.

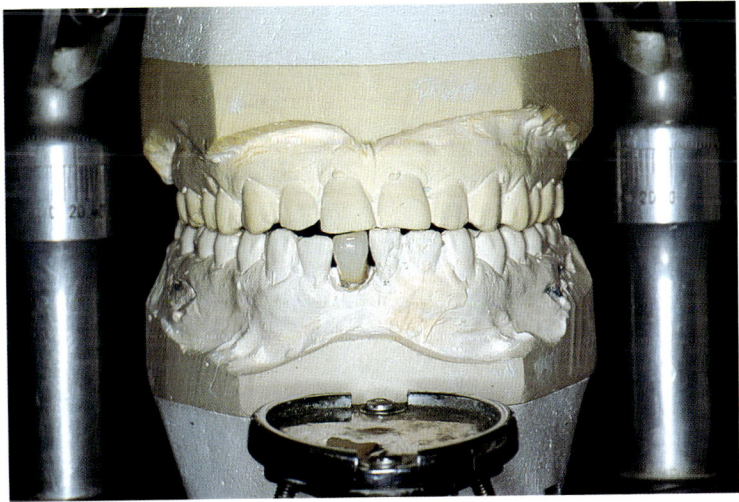

Fig 4-19 Slurrying and firing porcelain follows standard procedures. In the case shown, a narrow cervical margin will aid an aesthetic result.

fabricated sintered ceramic cylinder. In the system demonstrated the cylinder is manufactured from a gold alloy with a press fit waxing sheath (Fig 4-17), that is suitable for casting with the majority of precious and semi-precious bonding alloys (Fig 4-18), and a design which encourages a gradual increase in tooth bulk from the cervical margin (Fig 4-19). On the articulator it is necessary to check that the crown is in light contact (Shimstock®, Hanel-GMH-Dental, W. Germany) in occlusion and that it is free of premature or non-working side contacts. If the tooth being replaced is a canine, it is preferable to place the associated quadrant into group function, thus preventing overload of the implant in lateral excursions. If however the tooth is in any other position it is wise to opt for natural canine and/or anterior guidance so that the implant borne restoration is in discclusion during these excursive movements. An assessment of crown:implant ratio will also influence occlusal contact, since an unavoidably long crown, the result of excessive crestal bone loss, will lead to unfavourable moment arm forces, which may result in crown loosening or implant overload. In these cases it may be preferable to place the restoration out of contact in working excursions. Insertion of the crown is technically simple, using a standard cementation procedure (Fig 4-20). Prior to cementation it is necessary to protect the head of the abutment screw with some cotton wool or Fermit® (Ivoclar-Vivadent UK Ltd, England). Cement should be sparingly applied to both the inside of the crown and the abutment, preferably using a brush. The cement of choice should be Zinc Phosphate or Glass Ionomer for permanent cementation and a modified Temp Bond® (Kerr UK Ltd, England) for provisional cementation, which may be necessary if there are doubts about shade or crown contour. In all cases it is essential that an even pressure is applied and that the crown is correctly seated, fully engaging the external hexagon or octagon. The use of intra oral radiographs will confirm whether or not a crown is accurately seated (Fig 4-21 and 4-22).

There is little doubt, that the single tooth implant will do much to restore the dental imbalance of tooth loss and social embarrassment caused by anterior single tooth loss, without relying on the support or destruction of adjacent tissues (Fig 4-23 and 4-24).

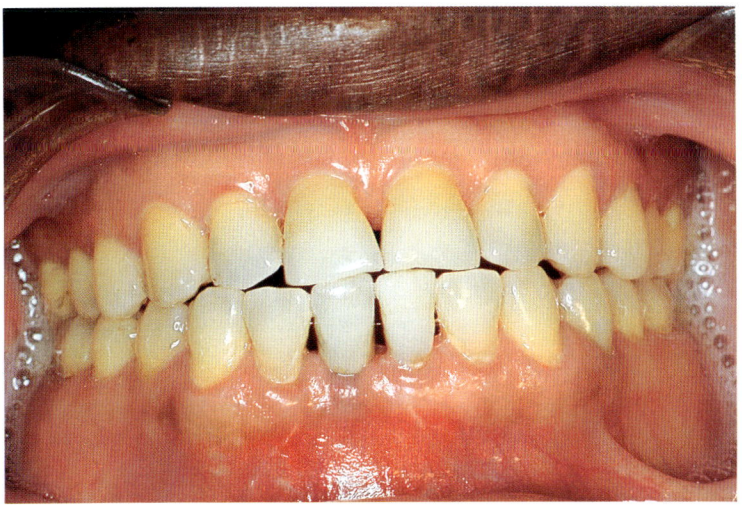

Fig 4-20 The crown is inserted and checked for aesthetics, occlusion and contact schemes. Permanent cementation is effected by the use of zinc phosphate, glass ionomer, or composite cements.

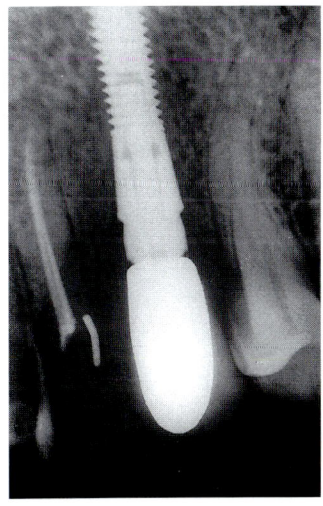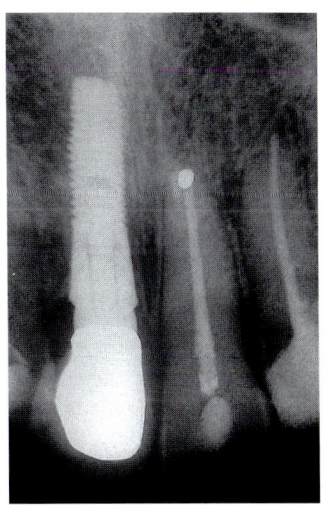

Fig 4-21   Fig 4-22

Fig 4-21 (left) The abutment design allows for an appreciation of accurate seating but post insertion radiographs are advisable to assess accuracy of fit. This canine is incorrectly positioned and will require removal and reseating.

Fig 4-22 (right) This radiograph of a central incisor shows the crown correctly cemented in place.

77

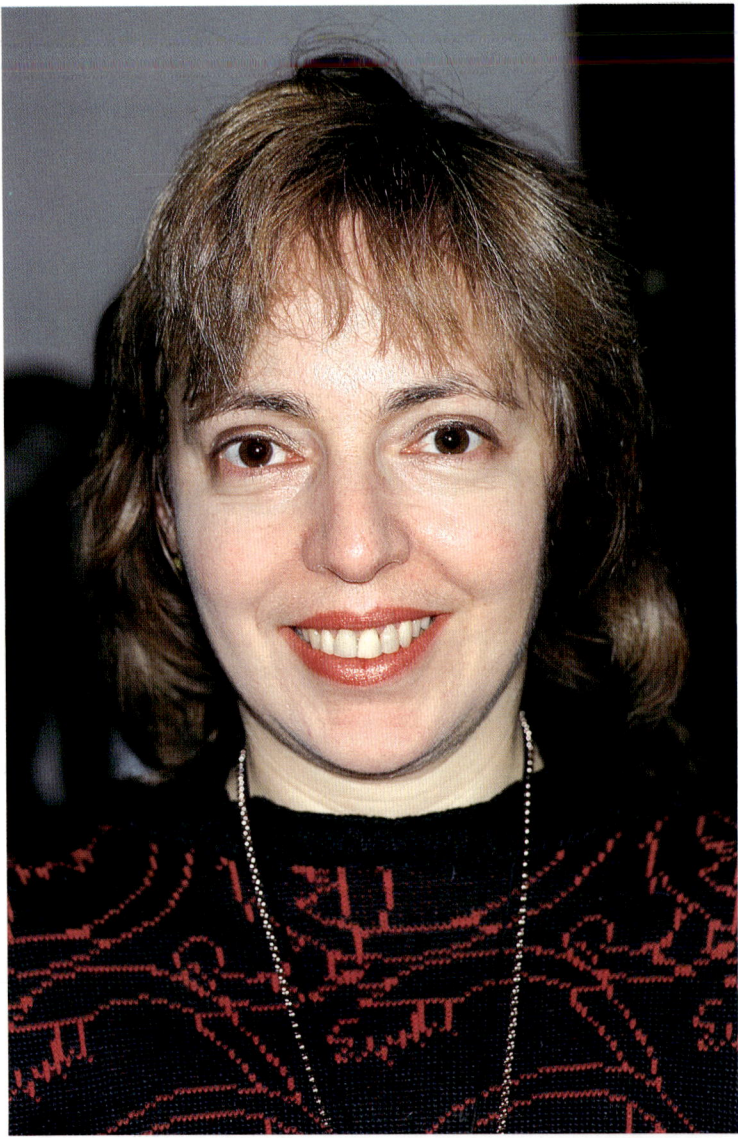

Fig 4-23 The overall effect of permanent tooth replacement, especially where there may have been social embarrassment, is profound and extends well beyond simple dental rehabilitation. With care and attention to soft tissues and the aesthetics of the ceramometal restoration (see fig 4-24), an implant retained crown can prove a most natural tooth replacement.

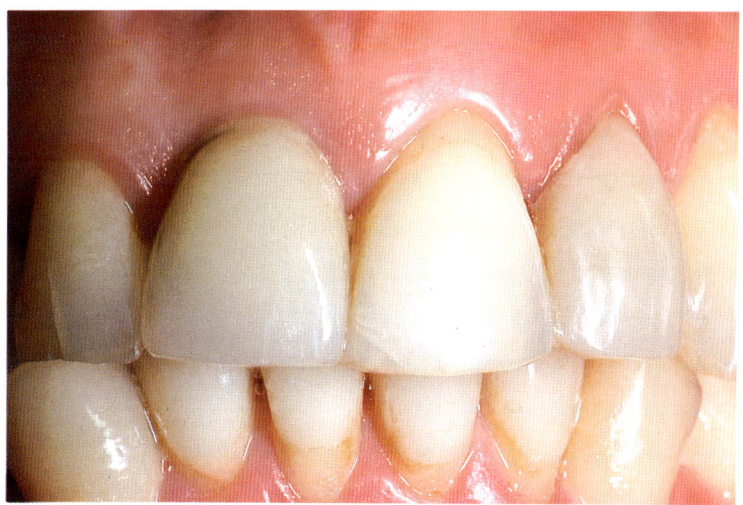

Fig 4-24 A close-up view of the restoration shown in fig 4-23.

References

1 *Balshi, T.* Implant esthetics. 2. Understand nature of tooth loss before tackling anterior maxillary single tooth replacement. Dent Implantol Update 1991; 2: 79-81.

2 *Lewis, S.G., Beumer III, J., Perri, G.R., Hornburg, W.P.* Single tooth implant supported restorations. Int J Oral Maxillofac Implants 1988; 3: 25-30.

3 *Schmitt, A., Zarb, G.A.* The longitudinal clinical effectiveness of osseointegrated dental implants for single-tooth replacement. Int J Prosthodont 1993; 6: 197-202.

4 *Scheerer, E.W., Wessberg, G.A.* Aesthetic restorations with Brånemark system: single-tooth replacements. Hawaii Dent J 1991; 22: 9-12.

5 *Jemt, T., Laney, W.R., Harris, D., Henry, P.J., Krogh, P.H. Jr., Polizzi, G., Zarb, G.A., Herrmann, I.* Osseointegrated implants for single tooth replacement: A 1-year report from a multicenter prospective study. Int J Oral Maxillofac Implants 1991; 6: 29-36.

6 *Sager, R.D., Thies, R.M.* Implant-retained precision two-stage single-tooth replacement. J Oral Implantol 1991; 17: 166-171.

7 *Rogoff, G.S.* A new step-by-step approach: CeraOne single-tooth replacement. Dent Implantol Update 1991; 2: 42-44.

8 *Andersson, B., Odman, P., Carlsson, L., Brånemark, P.-I.* A new Brånemark single tooth abutment: handling and early clinical experiences. Int J Oral Maxillofac Implants 1992; 7: 105-111.

9 *Patrick, D.R., Dorfman, W.M.* Achieving anterior aesthetics with an anti-rotational abutment. Pract Periodontics Aesthet Dent 1992; 4: 13-16.

10 *Lewis, S.G., Llamas, D., Avera, A.* The UCLA abutment: a four-year review. J Prosthet Dent 1992; 67: 509-515.

11 *Jaggers, A., Simons, A.M., Badr, S.E.* Abutment selection for anterior single tooth replacement. A clinical report. J Prosthet Dent 1993; 69: 133-135.

12 *Gotfredsen, K., Nimb, L., Hjörting-Hansen, E., Jensen, J.S., Holmén, A.* Histomorphometric and removal torque analysis for TiO_2-blasted titanium implants. Clin Oral Impl Res 1992; 3: 77-84.

13 *Ericsson, I., Johansson, C.B., Bystedt, H., Norton, M.R.* A histomorphometric evaluation of bone to implant contact on machine prepared and roughened titanium dental implants. Clin Oral Impl Res 1994; 5: 202-206.

14 *Schroeder, A., Pohler, O., Sutter, F.* Gewebereaktion auf ein Titan-Hohlzylinderimplantat mit Titan-Spritzschichtoberfläche. Schweiz Mschr Zahnheilk 1976; 86: 713-727.

15 *Schroeder, A., van der Zypen, E., Stich, H., Sutter, F.* The reaction of bone, connective tissue and epithelium to endosteal implants with sprayed titanium surfaces. J Maxillofac Surg 1981; 9: 15-25.

16 *Cook, S.D., Kay, J.F., Thomas, K.A., Jarcho, M.* Interface mechanics and histology of titanium and hydroxylapatite-coated titanium for dental implant applications. Int J Oral Maxillofac Implants 1987; 2: 15-22.

17 *Cook, S.D., Baffes, G.C., Thomas, K.A.* Comparison of models for evaluating interface characteristics of HA-coated implants. J Dent Res 1991; 70: 530. Abstract 2115.

18 *Buser, D.A., Schroeder, A. Sutter, F., Lang, N.P.* The new concept of ITI hollow-cylinder and hollow-screw implants: Part 2. Clinical aspects, indications, and early clinical results. Int J Oral Maxillofac Implants 1988; 3: 173-181.

5 Fixed Bridge Rehabilitation (FBR)

The earliest Brånemark studies,[1-3] dealing with FBR, all concentrated on the provision of full arch prostheses, principally in the mandible, screw retained to six titanium implants placed between the mental foramina. In these early cases, great care was taken in selecting ideal candidates and constructing bridges that were essentially functional, retrievable and hygienic. Such parameters lent themselves to a bridge design that has subsequently been labelled the "oil rig" or "high water line" prosthesis (Fig 5-1).

These bridges were generally fabricated from gold alloys with acrylic teeth and gum work mechanically bonded to the metalwork and with adequate space left available between the bridge and the mucosa to allow access for effective oral hygiene. Two premolar units were usually cantilevered distal to the most distal implant to restore adequate arch form and bridge screw access (that is the screws that retained the bridge to the abutments), was facilitated through access holes in the occlusal surfaces of the teeth.

Many of these prostheses have 25+ years of success in function and are still in place today. However it is only as a result of the twenty years ongoing research that we are able to begin to understand why these bridges work and what the causes are when they fail. Such research and anecdotal clinical findings have also continued to reshape our clinical viewpoint as to what is feasible, recognising that perhaps implants would have a much wider use in the partially dentate patient, particularly in restoring the type of dentitions as described by the Kennedy Applegate classification.

It is not possible to cover all of the extensive information that has arisen from studies of full and partial reconstruction with dental implants, though the literature has an abundance of reports pertaining to various implants and their success,[4-16] most of which present details on prosthetic techniques specific to the implant system and area for reconstruction. However, peripheral research on implant supported bridgework has also done much to educate the prosthodontist as to what is permissible

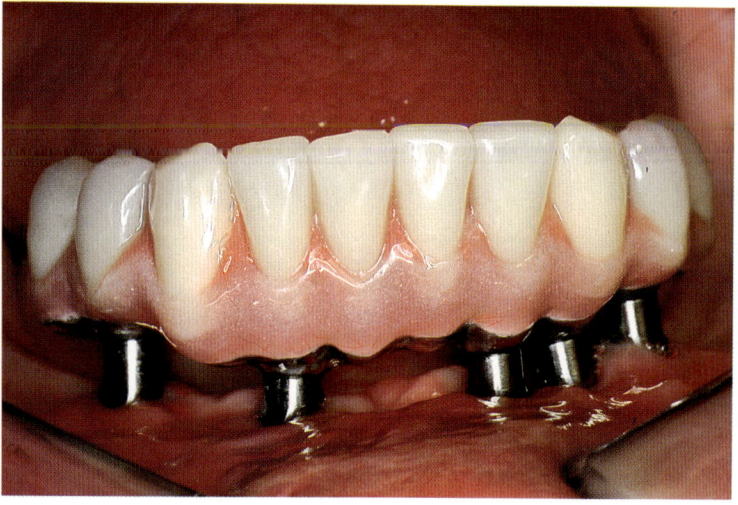

Fig 5-1 The "oil rig" or "high water line" prosthesis satisfies many requirements, particularly for mandibular reconstruction, but has proven less popular due to limitations of aesthetics and phonetics.

in implant retained FBR. Most of this peripheral work concentrated on bite force,[17-22] chewing patterns and efficiency,[22-26] muscle function[27] and occlusal perception.[28]

Data collated from these studies is incontrovertible in confirming that implant supported bridgework restores oral function and bite force to a level approaching that of patients with natural teeth and achieves levels of occlusal perception at the $50\mu m$ level compared to $100\mu m$ for conventional dentures and $20\mu m$ for natural teeth.[28]

Loading and Stress Distribution

The work of Professor Skalak[29] in 1983 also instigated new avenues of thought as he introduced concepts of biomechanics into an otherwise clinical arena. His much quoted work analysed the forces imparted to each implant within a fixed bridge system, highlighting the profound influence that implant numbers, inter implant distance and cantilever distance all have on the distribution of occlusal and lateral loads; as also does the shape and quality of the metal framework.[30]

The study of complex loading and stress distribution within implant supported fixed bridgework was extended to the use of finite element analysis, [31-33] using a computer assisted method, by which a system can be compartmentalised into many smaller elements. This enables the effects of an applied force to be measured within the system as a whole; within collective units, or within single elements. Such studies have given valuable insight into the cause and effect of using various casting alloys and have educated us with respect to maximum cantilever length;[33] and, in particular, have compared the use of acrylic resin to porcelain occlusal surfaces.[32]

From computer assisted predictions it has been possible to progress to measure load and stress distribution within *in vivo* FBR systems[34] and record the effects of varying occlusal materials on the load distribution to the supporting framework.[35] This is made possible through the use of force transducers and strain gauges. Perhaps the greatest of links between this research and clinical practice is the recent report of a special interactive software package based on the Skalak model, which allows computer aided design of prostheses based on patient bite force, number of fixtures, fixture co-ordinates, and direction of applied forces, the details of which can be input by the use of special grids and measurements.[36]

The reader is directed to the references at the end of the chapter for details of those articles which will provide the necessary further reading since it should be stressed that in such an introductory text, details of the findings of these studies is strictly limited to basic concepts.

Prosthesis Fabrication

The basic protocol for prosthesis fabrication is similar amongst the various systems, though again the reader would be wise to seek details of individual protocols for their system of choice.

Selecting Final Abutments

Chapter 3 has already addressed the various methods for assessing abutment length and the technique used to insert final abutments. In the Astra system it is recommended that 20° abutments are selected when considering reconstruction with fixed bridgework; the substantial vertical component of the conus providing adequate support for the prosthesis against lateral loads and hence protecting the small bridge screw.

Impression Techniques

Advantage should be taken of pre-fabricated impression copings which are screwed to the abutments. The direct or squared impression copings are secured to the abutments by means of a central guide pin, which remains exposed during the impression taking, through windows cut in to the customised impression tray (Fig 5-2).

The tray windows are covered with soft wax to keep the impression

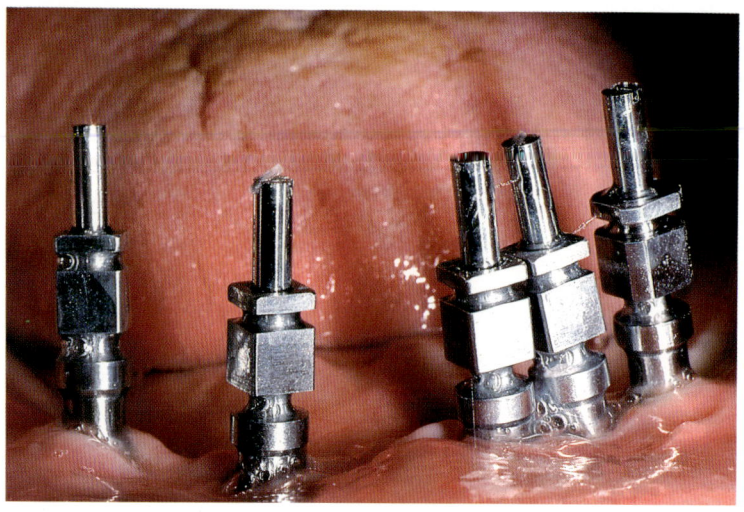

Fig 5-2 Direct or "squared" impression copings are secured to abutments by means of central screws or guide pins. Access windows are incorporated into the customised tray to facilitate unscrewing of guide pins, to allow impression withdrawal.

material, which should ideally be Impregum® or a material of similar properties, from oozing out. On final set, it is now possible to gain access to the guide pins which are unscrewed. The impression can now be withdrawn with the squared copings remaining *in situ* (Fig 5-3). Such a technique ensures the accurate position and relation of each coping within the impression. Clearly impression definition is of importance, but retention of copings and their relation to each other is the most critical aspect, with peripheral details perhaps less important than with conventional impressions.

Unfortunately, it is not always practical to get copings, impression tray,

guide pins, screwdriver, and hand all in the patient's mouth and it is therefore necessary to sometimes use an indirect technique with tapered copings (Fig 5-4). These are screwed directly to the implants and remain so on withdrawal of the impression. It is then necessary to unscrew each coping, replacing it firmly in to its respective site in the impression. Though it would seem that such a technique can not guarantee the accurate reproduction of position and relation of each coping within the impression, studies have in fact shown it to be as good as the direct technique.[42, 43]

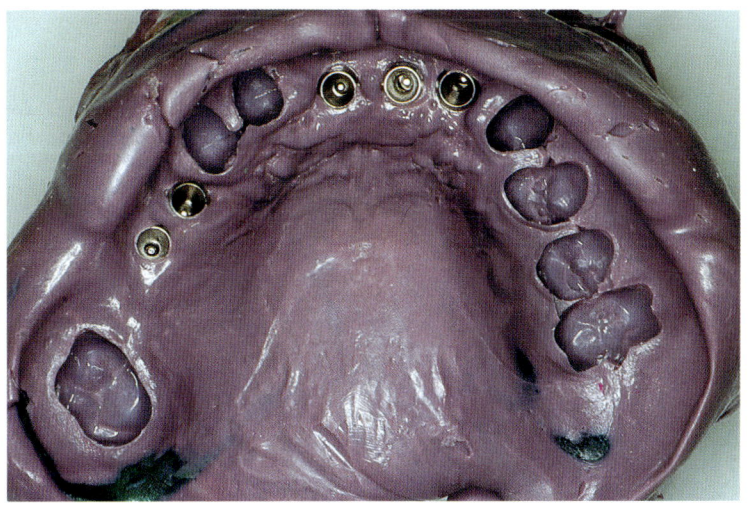

Fig 5-3 Direct impression copings are so-called, because they remain *in situ* on withdrawal of the impression.

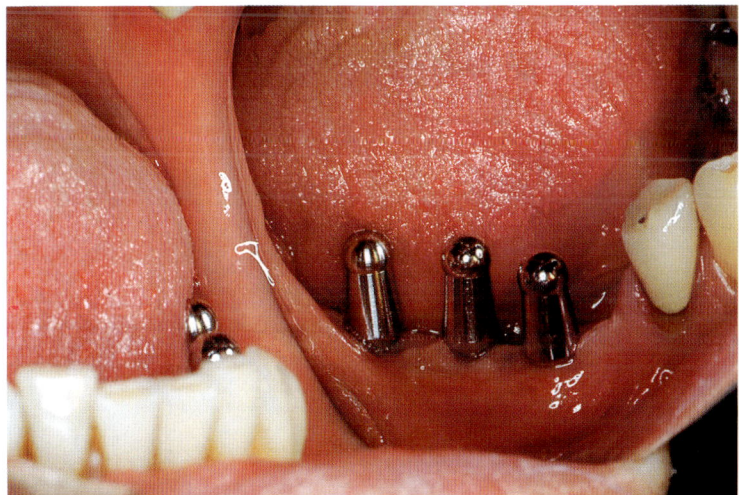

Fig 5-4 Indirect or "tapered" impression copings screw directly on to the abutments. On withdrawal of the impression, these copings need to be unscrewed from the abutments and reseated in the impression.

The result of all these studies can be generalised as follows:

1   The greater the number of implants available to support a fixed bridge, the more favourable the load distribution.
2   Implants should ideally be placed to receive axial loading in preference to non axial loading.
3   When three or more implants are placed, it is preferable that they be just offset from a strictly linear arrangement.
4   Cantilevers should be kept to a maximum length of 12mm.
5   Occlusal table width should be reduced, whilst maintaining an axial load.
6   Never place both mesial and distal cantilevers on a bridge supported by only two implants.
7   The use of ceramometal for prosthetic restorations does not appear to be contraindicated as first thought.

To further confound the clinician, the above principles only govern a fixed bridge constructed on osseointegrated implants. The controversial topic of joining teeth to implants introduces even more complex issues of combining essentially ankylosed units with those that possess an inherent damping or shock absorbing system, the periodontal ligament. It was postulated that a bridge constructed on anchorage units of such a differing reslience would lead to biomechanical breakdown. Indeed one system, the IMZ system (Friatec

AG, Mannheim, Germany) incorporates a shock absorbing *intramobile element* or IME between fixture and abutment, which acts to dissipate occlusal load during function.[37-39] Not all studies have borne out the findings of the IME[40] whilst some studies have shown equally good success rates when using other implant systems in partial reconstruction's joining teeth to implants.[41] However it may be that for the novice, an eighth rule should apply:

8   It is desirable that implants and teeth should not be combined in an FBR if at all possible.

Some systems, such as the ITI system (Institute Straumann AG, Waldenburg, Switzerland) offer the option to work on abutments, to which a conventional type bridge is directly cemented. For such systems, standard impressions of the abutments are taken as if they were conventional preparations and bridgework is fabricated on stone dies.

In an effort to achieve manufacturer precision in the mouth, the use of impression copings directly implicates the use of prefabricated abutment replicas which are screwed to the copings prior to casting (Fig 5 - 5). This allows the technician to fabricate the bridgework on metal dies (abutment replicas) incorporated into the master cast (Fig 5 - 6), rather than on stone dies.

It is now possible to construct bite blocks, temporary bridgework, and final bridgework on prefabricated

invaluable, should it be required at a later date, if for any reason the permanent bridge has to be removed.

Final Bridge Fabrication

Having satisfied all of the above concerns with a transitional prosthesis, one is now in a strong position to proceed with final bridge fabrication. Clearly the fit of the transitional prosthesis is an indication of the accuracy of the master cast though not a guarantee, but it should be a sound basis for using the same working cast for final bridge construction.

The metal framework will likely be constructed around prefabricated gold alloy cylinders that relate precisely to the geometry of the abutment and abutment replica. Cylinders are screwed to the replica by means of a bridge screw and the wax up (Fig 5-11), which incorporates each cylinder into the eventual framework, is cast in precious or semi-precious bonding alloys.

Frameworks will vary according to the type of prosthesis to be fabricated. For the type of screw retained restorations being presented in this chapter, there are essentially two alternatives. The strictly *ad modum* Brånemark screw retrievable bridge will present a framework that is splinted as a single unit (Fig 5-12): whereby each bridge screw will contribute to the overall fixation of the bridge, with porcelain being fired directly to the framework. In this scenario it is possible to remove the bridge screws through access holes in the occlusal surfaces of the bridge (Fig 5-13).

The alternative concept is termed double construction, and is based on the principle of cementing a superstructure to individual screw retained copings or to a splinted substructure. The individual copings (Fig 5-12: maxilla) and the splinted substructure (Fig 5-14) are both fabricated around the same precision fit bridge cylinders, so that they locate accurately to both the abutment replica and the abutment and are secured with the bridge screws.

In order to relate the position of individual copings from the master cast to the mouth, it is essential to use an acrylic template which will maintain their position during the transfer (Fig 5-15). On securing the copings, it is then possible to slip off the transfer template (Fig 5-16).

The superstructure is then fabricated in the laboratory to accurately fit over the substructure with a small cementation space. The value of such a double construction is that it is possible to achieve a more aesthetically pleasing result with the absence of occlusal access holes (Fig 5-17a and b). Also it has the ability to correct inclination problems by means of waxing the subcopings back into the arch line, thus avoiding the use of angulated abutments.

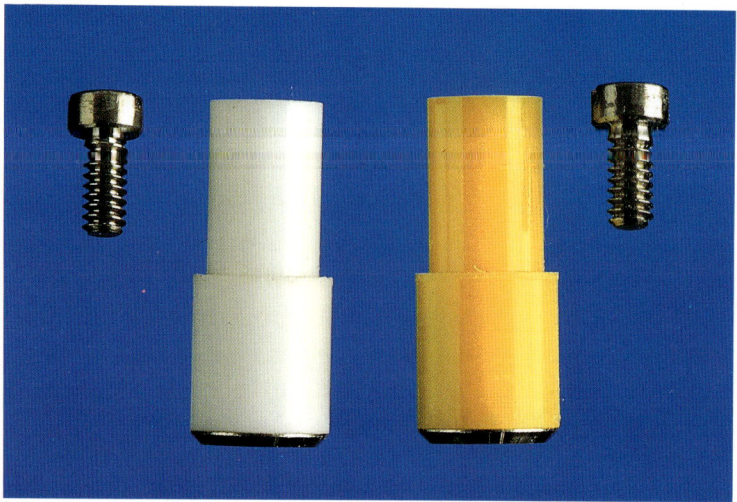

Fig 5-11 Framework wax-up incorporates precision fit, prefabricated, gold alloy bridge cylinders, which are encased in a plastic waxing sheath. These semi-burnout cylinders have a melting point of 1450°C and can be cast with most precious and semi precious bonding alloys.

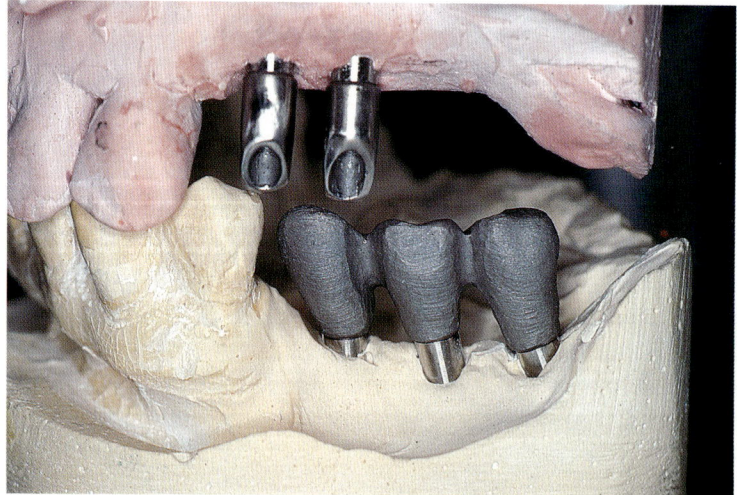

Fig 5-12 Mandible: The cast framework splints all three implants. Porcelain will be fired directly to this metal framework, which will be a screw retrievable prosthesis.

Maxilla: Individual sub-copings have been cast and are secured separately to their respective abutments. A porcelain fused to metal bridge will subsequently be fabricated to cement over the top as part of a double construction.

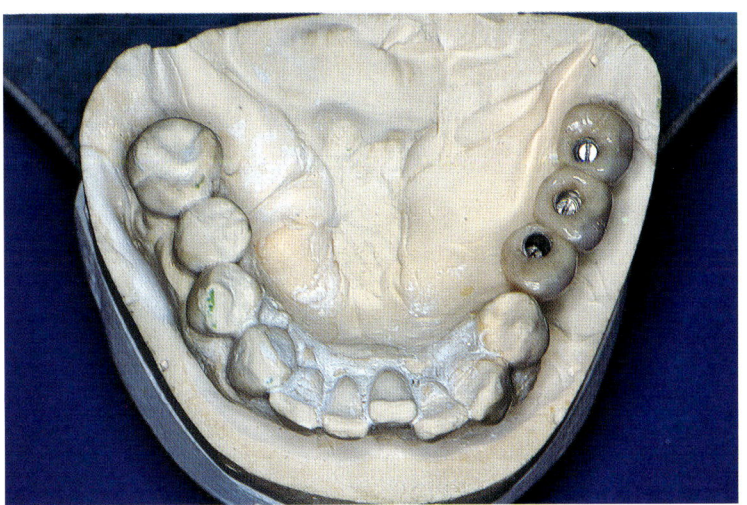

Fig 5-13 Access to bridge screws is facilitated through the occlusal surfaces of the screw retrievable bridge. Access holes are eventually occluded with light cured composite.

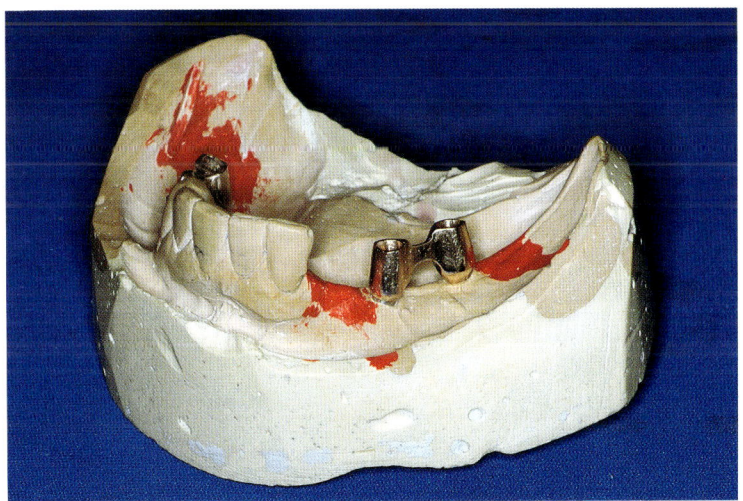

Fig 5-14 When opting for the double construction, it is possible to splint the sub copings for additional support of shorter implants.

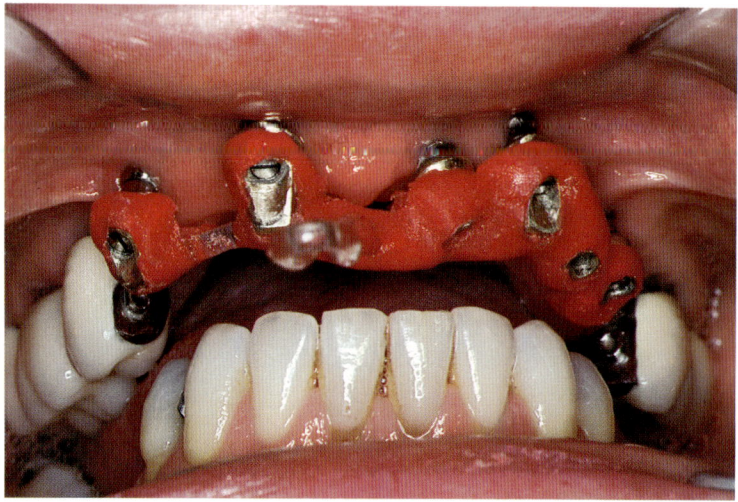

Fig 5-15 In order to transfer multiple copings from the master cast to the mouth, a transfer template is fabricated in resin, splinting copings in their correct positions.

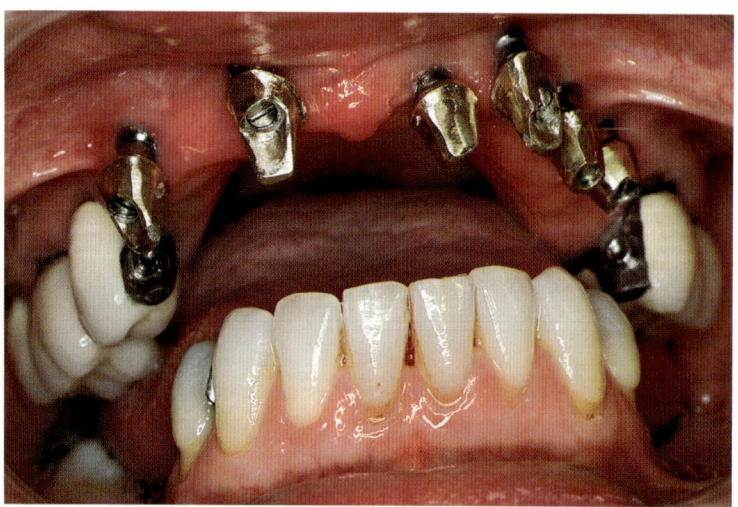

Fig 5-16 On tightly securing all copings to their respective abutments, it is possible to slip the transfer template off. Bridge copings remain in the correct orientation for subsequent cementation of the superstructure.

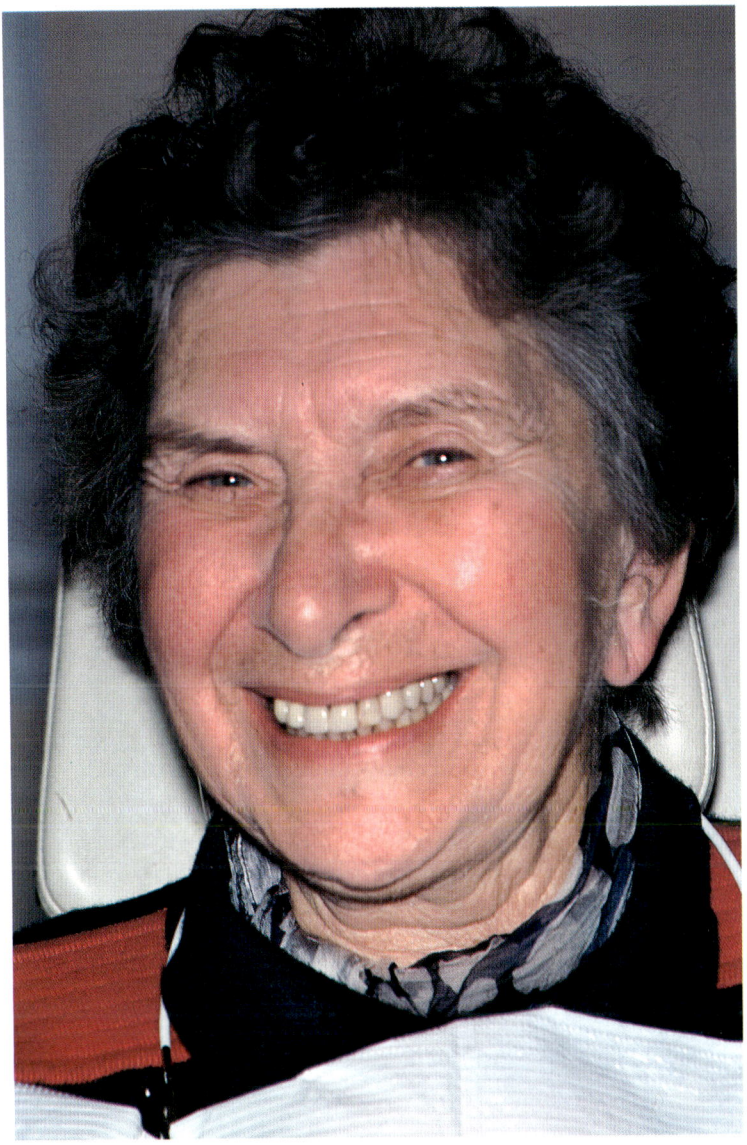

Fig 5-21 Assessment of aesthetics, though important to the clinician, is the right of the patient. It is well worth remembering that a bridge that satisfies all criteria, except for patient satisfaction of aesthetics, is doomed to failure.

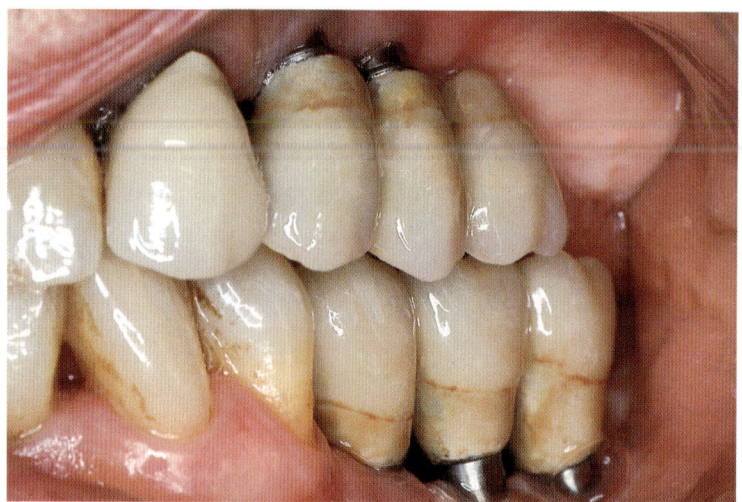

Fig 5-22 Light contact in centric should be assessed by means of Shimstock™ and articulating paper. It is important that all implant supported prostheses also demonstrate axial loading in centric, if possible.

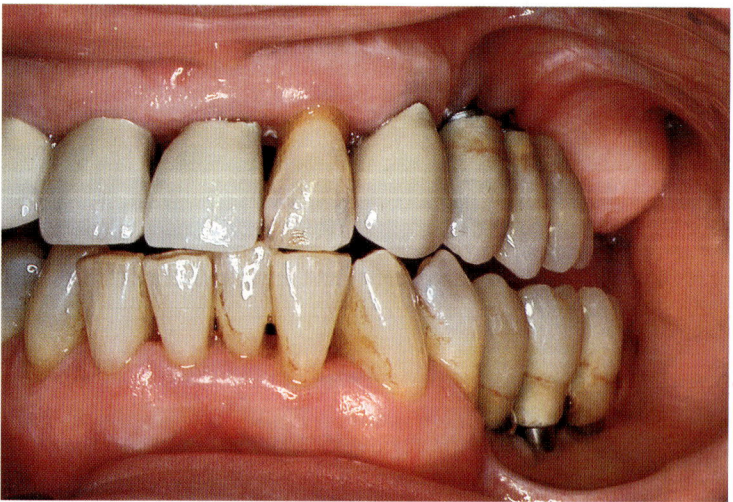

Fig 5-23 An assessment of working side contacts should demonstrate a balanced distribution of load and excursive movements should always demonstrate canine guidance in the presence of a natural canine, or group function when the canine is incorporated into the implant restoration.

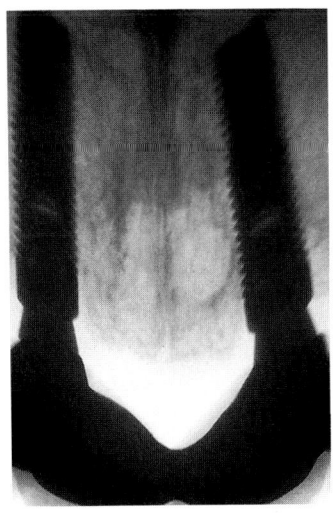

Fig 5-24 A one year post insertion radiograph of this anterior implant retained double construction clearly demonstrates a propitious crestal bone level. In the absence of clinical signs, this would suggest a satisfactory bridge design, with favourable load distribution to the supporting implants.

Table 5-1   Occlusal Factors for Clinical Assessment

1   The demonstration of light cusp/fossa contact in centric.
2   The presence of balanced working side contacts.
3   The absence of premature and non-working side contacts.
4   The absence of interferences during excursive movements.
5   Canine guidance, when in the presence of a natural canine.
6   Group function, when in the absence of a natural canine.

An intra-oral assessment of the occlusion should be undertaken with the use of Shimstock™ and articulating paper. An appraisal of conventional occlusal factors (Table 5-1) are applied to the implant retained FBR. Clearly the paramount requisite is that the implants should be loaded in an axial manner, with an even distribution of occlusal forces. Lateral and shear forces are to be avoided as these represent a potential threat to all levels of the bone-implant-masticatory complex.

An assessment of aesthetics is as always in the eye of the patient. However in an effort to achieve the ideal, it is often invaluable if the patient can provide an old photograph that clearly demonstrates their own natural dentition, prior to its demise, so that the ceramist has a firm idea of how the end result should appear.

Recall appointments should be made at 1 week and 1 month post insertion. One will often find a number of complaints after the first week, particularly when a patient has been converted from a conventional denture to fixed bridgework. These usually follow a format of poor speech control, food impaction and poor control of salivary flow. Reassurance will often suffice and indeed second recall usually confirms that many of these adaptive problems have subsided.

According to some protocols it may also be necessary at first recall to gain access to bridge screws to re-tighten them. Experience with the Astra system has shown this to be a rare requirement, though it is advisable to always assess mobility of the bridge.

Subsequent recall structure should follow a six monthly or annual visit, with a hygiene appointment booked alongside the review. In this way it is possible to monitor the implant retained FBR. Radiographs should be taken on an annual basis to allow monitoring of the crestal bone level (Fig 5-24) and the bone/implant interface.

References

1 *Adell, R., Lekholm, U., Rockler, B., Bråne-mark, P.-I.* A 15-year study of osseointe-grated implants in the treatment of the edentulous jaw. Int J Oral Surg 1981; 10: 387-416.

2 *Brånemark, P.-I., Hansson, B.O., Adell, R., Breine, U., Lindström, J., Hallen, O., Öhman, A.* Osseointegrated implants in the treat-ment of the edentulous jaw. Experience from a 10-year period. Scand J Plast Reconstr Surg 1977; 11: Suppl 16.

3 *Adell, R.* Clinical results of osseointegrated implants supporting fixed prostheses in edentulous jaws. J Prosthet Dent 1983; 50: 251-254.

4 *Lundqvist, S., Carlsson, G.E.* Maxillary fixed prostheses on osseointegrated dental im-plants. J Prosthet Dent 1983; 50: 262-270.

5 *Jemt, T.* Modified single and short-span restorations supported by osseointegrated fixtures in the partially edentulous jaw. J Prosthet Dent 1986; 55: 243-247.

6 *Cox, J.F., Zarb, G.A.* The longitudinal clinical efficacy of osseointegrated dental implants: A 3-year report. Int J Oral Maxil-lofac Implants 1987; 2: 91-100.

7 *Jones, S.D., Jones, F.R.* Tissue-integrated implants for the partially edentulous patient. J Prosthet Dent 1988; 60: 349-354.

8 *Zarb, G.A., Schmitt, A.* The longitudinal clinical effectiveness of osseointegrated dental implants: The Toronto study. Part II: The prosthetic results. J Prosthet Dent 1990; 64: 53-61.

9 *Jemt, T., Lekholm, U., Adell, R.* Osseointe-grated implants in the treatment of partially edentulous patients: A preliminary study on 876 consecutively placed fixtures. Int J Oral Maxillofac Implants 1989; 4: 211-217.

10 *Tzakis, M.G., Linden, B., Jemt, T.* Oral function in patients treated with prostheses on Brånemark osseointegrated implants in partially edentulous jaws: A pilot study. Int J Oral Maxillofac Implants 1990; 5: 107-111.

11 *Buser, D., Weber, H.P., Brägger, U., Balsiger, C.* Tissue integration of one-stage ITI im-plants: 3-year results of a longitudinal study with hollow-cylinder and hollow-screw implants. Int J Oral Maxillofac Implants 1991; 6: 405-412.

12 *Arvidson, K., Bystedt, H., Frykholm, A., von Konow, L. Lothigius, E.* A 3-year clinical study of Astra dental implants in the treat-ment of edentulous mandibles. Int J Oral Maxillofac Implants 1992; 7: 321-329.

13 *Zarb, G.A., Schmitt, A.* The longitudinal clinical effectiveness of osseointegrated dental implants in anterior partially eden-tulous patients. Int J Prosthodont 1993; 6: 180-188.

14 *Zarb, G.A., Schmitt, A.* The longitudinal clinical effectiveness of osseointegrated dental implants in posterior partially eden-tulous patients. Int J Prosthodont 1993; 6: 189-196.

15 *Babbush, C.A., Shimura, M.* Five-year statis-tical and clinical observations with the IMZ two-stage osseointegrated implant system. Int J Oral Maxillofac Implants 1993; 8: 245-253.

16 *Stultz, E.R., Lofland, R., Sendax, V.I., Horn-buckle, C.* A multicentre 5 year retrospec-tive survival analysis of 6200 Integral® im-plants. Comp Continuing Educ 1993; 14: 478-486.

17 *Haraldson, T., Carlsson, G.E.* Bite force and oral function in patients with osseo-integrated oral implants. Scand J Dent Res 1977; 85: 200-208.

18 *Haraldson, T., Carlsson, G.E., Ingervall, B.* Functional state, bite force and postural muscle activity in patients with osseointe-grated oral implant bridges. Acta Odontol Scand 1979; 37: 195-206.

19 *Carr, A.B., Laney, W.R.* Maximum occlusal force levels in patients with osseointe-grated oral implant prostheses and patients with complete dentures. Int J Oral Maxillofac Implants 1987; 2: 101-108.

20 *Falk, H., Laurell, L., Lundgren, D.* Occlusal force pattern in dentitions with mandibular implant-supported fixed cantilever pros-theses occluded with complete dentures. Int J Oral Maxillofac Implants 1989; 4: 55-62.

21 *Falk, H., Laurell, L., Lundgren, D.* Occlusal interferences and cantilever joint stress in implant-supported prostheses occluding with complete dentures. Int J Oral Maxil-lofac Implants 1990; 5: 70-77.

22 Lundqvist, S., Haraldson, T. Oral function in patients wearing fixed prosthesis on osseointegrated implants in the maxilla: 3-year follow-up study. Scand J Dent Res 1992; 100: 279-283.

23 Haraldson, T., Carlsson, G.E. Chewing efficacy in patients with osseointegrated oral implant bridges. Swed Dent J 1979; 3: 183-191.

24 Jemt, T., Lindquist, L., Hedegård, B. Changes in chewing patterns of patients with complete dentures after placement of osseointegrated implants in the mandible. J Prosthet Dent 1985; 53: 578-583.

25 Lindquist, L.W., Carlsson, G.E. Long-term effects on chewing with mandibular fixed prostheses on osseointegrated implants. Acta Odontol Scand 1985; 43: 39-45.

26 Lindquist, L.W., Carlsson, G.E. Changes in masticatory function in complete denture wearers after insertion of bridges on osseointegrated implants in the lower jaw. In: Clinical applications of biomaterials (eds Lee, A.J.C., Albrektsson, T., Brånemark, P.-I.), New York: John Wiley & Sons Inc., 1982.

27 Haraldson, T., Ingervall, B. Muscle function during chewing and swallowing in patients with osseointegrated oral implant bridges. An electromyographic study. Acta Odontol Scand 1979; 37: 207-216.

28 Lundqvist, S., Haraldson, T. Occlusal perception of thickness in patients with bridges on osseointegrated oral implants. Scand J Dent Res 1984; 92: 88-92.

29 Skalak, R. Biomechanical considerations in osseointegrated prostheses. J Prosthet Dent 1983; 49: 843-849.

30 Brunski, J.B., Skalak, R. Biomechanics of osseointegration and dental prostheses. In: Osseointegration in oral rehabilitation (eds Naert, I., van Steenberghe, D., Worthington, P.), pp 133-156. Berlin: Quintessence, 1993.

31 Davis, D.M., Zarb, G.A., Chao, Y-L. Studies on frameworks for osseointegrated prostheses: Part 1. The effect of varying the number of supporting abutments. Int J Oral Maxillofac Implants 1988; 3: 197-201.

32 Davis, D.M., Rimrott, R., Zarb, G.A. Studies on frameworks for osseointegrated prostheses: Part 2. The effect of adding acrylic resin or porcelain to form the occlusal superstructure. Int J Oral Maxillofac Implants 1988; 3: 275-280.

33 Williams, K.R., Watson, C.J., Murphy, W.M., Scott, J., Gregory, M., Sinobad, D. Finite element analysis of fixed prostheses attached to osseointegrated implants. Quintessence Int 1990; 21: 563-570.

34 Jemt, T., Carlsson, L. Boss, A. Jörnéus, L. In vivo load measurements on osseointegrated implants supporting fixed or removable prostheses: A comparative pilot study. Int J Oral Maxillofac Implants 1991; 6: 413-417.

35 Hobkirk, J.A., Psarros, K.J. The influence of occlusal surface material on peak masticatory forces using osseointegrated implant-supported prostheses. Int J Oral Maxillofac Implants 1992; 7: 345-352.

36 Monteith, B.D. Minimising biomechanical overload in implant prostheses: A computerised aid to design. J Prosthet Dent 1993; 69: 495-502.

37 Kirsch, A., Ackerman, K.L. The IMZ osseointegrated implant system. Dent Clin North Am 1989; 33: 733-761.

38 Chapman, R.J., Kirsch, A. Variations in occlusal forces with resilient internal implant shock absorber. Int J Oral Maxillofac Implants 1990; 5: 369-374.

39 Kay, H.B. Free-standing versus implant-tooth-interconnected restorations: Understanding the prosthodontic perspective. Int J Periodont Rest Dent 1993; 13: 47-69.

40 Holmes, D.C., Grigsby, W.R., Goel, V.K., Keller, J.C. Comparison of stress transmission in the IMZ implant system with polyoxymethylene or titanium intramobile element: A finite element stress analysis. Int J Oral Maxillofac Implants 1992; 7: 450-458.

41 Åstrand, P., Borg, K., Gunne, J., Olsson, M. Combination of natural teeth and osseointegrated implants as prosthesis abutments: A 2-year longitudinal study. Int J Oral Maxillofac Implants 1991; 6: 305-312.

42 Spector, M.R., Donovan, T.E., Nicholls, J.I. An evaluation of impression techniques for osseointegrated implants. J Prosthet Dent 1990; 63: 444-447.

43 Carr, A.B. Comparison of impression techniques for a two-implant 15-degree divergent model. Int J Oral Maxillofac Implants 1992; 7: 468-475.

6 Precision Attachments — Hybrid Fixed-Detachable Prosthesis

Experience with maxillary fixed prostheses over the last 15 years has drawn attention to a number of problems which arise as a direct result of the distopalatal atrophy of the maxilla, leading to poor implant orientation and inclination, and loss of lip support.

The subsequent prosthesis is often cantilevered labially to restore soft tissue support, with an attendant compromise of aesthetics and phonetics as air and saliva escape through the gaps between the bridge and the residual alveolus.

The need therefore exists for an alternative treatment therapy which would provide patients with the occlusal stability and retention of a fixed prosthesis, whilst restoring lip support and optimising conditions for phonetics and oral hygiene at the same time.

In 1991, Lothigius et al[1][2] published a two part article which presented the technical and clinical aspects of a new hybrid prosthesis with a design that incorporated separate support derived from a milled bar with lateral stabilisation obtained by a removable, close fitting, chrome based

prosthesis and retention provided by the incorporation of precision attachments. Such prostheses have been followed up successfully for two years and have a reported implant success rate comparable to maxillary fixed bridge prostheses.[3]

It was proposed that the design of the hybrid prosthesis would present the following features:

1 To splint the implants with the same rigidity as a fixed prosthesis.
2 Avoid palatal coverage, as compared to an overdenture.
3 Provide adequate lip support.
4 Optimise conditions for phonetics.
5 Facilitate oral hygiene procedures.
6 Provide adequate retention.
7 Incorporate serviceable precision attachments.

The original articles describe a horseshoe shaped overdenture, reinforced by a cast cobalt-chromium (Co/Cr) framework (Fig 6-1), which closely fits over a parallel sided

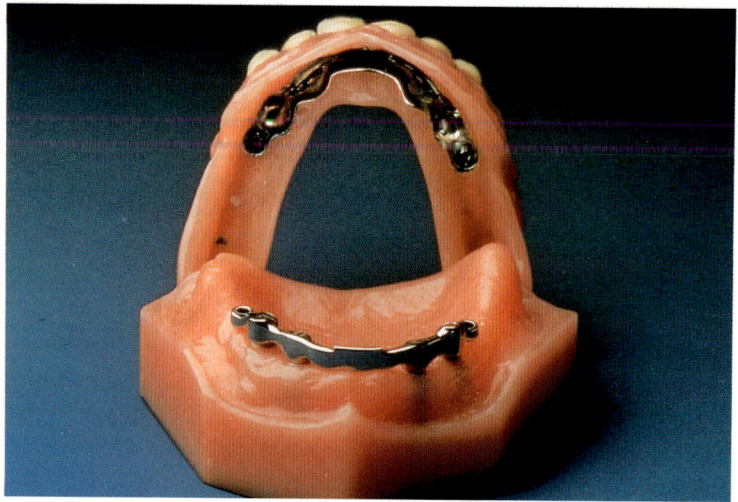

Fig 6-1 The hybrid prosthesis comprises a standard horseshoe denture which is reinforced with a cast Cobalt/Chromium framework, that is close fitting to the milled bar and incorporates the Ceka Revax (Ceka NV, Antwerp, Belgium) precision attachments.

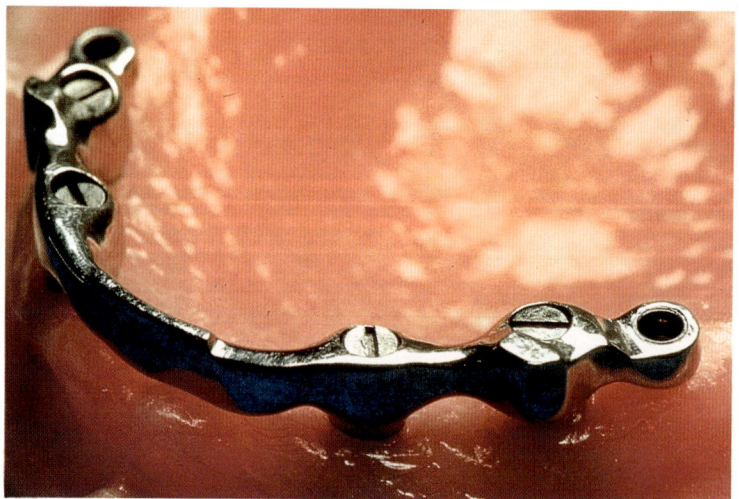

Fig 6-2 The milled bar is cast in a Type III dental gold alloy and is parallel sided to enhance lateral stability. Support for the overdenture is derived from the elevated areas of the bar. Female keepers are incorporated into the distal extensions which in combination with the patrix, provide the necessary retention.

milled bar, thus attaining support. Retention is derived from Ceka Revax attachments (Ceka NV, Antwerp, Belgium) which locate into the matrix incorporated at the distal ends of the milled bar (Fig 6-2). Lateral stabilisation is provided by the denture coverage, in particular over the tuberosities, and the labial flange ensures both adequate lip support and the prevention of air and salivary leakage.

In being a removable prosthesis, the requirement for hygiene maintenance is satisfied with direct access to the supporting implant substructure. In retrospect it is clear that the indications for use of a hybrid prosthesis may encompass a wide range of otherwise complex restorative cases, which can be identified by their mutual need to accommodate the following criteria:

1   Replacement of lost hard tissue support.
2   Replacement of lost soft tissue support.
3   The presence of an unfavourable ridge morphology.
4   The presence of unfavourably oriented and inclined implants.
5   The need to restore occlusal stability to a level approaching that of a fixed bridge prosthesis.

When considering the above, it is clear that a variety of developmental and acquired conditions might benefit from such a reconstruction, such as cleft palate patients and patients who have lost substantial hard tissues through trauma.

Case Presentation

The involvement of dental and alveolar trauma in accidents and assaults is not uncommon. The predisposition of the jaws to trauma often presents the restorative dentist with many problems as multiple teeth may be avulsed and require replacement. Restoration by means of conventional fixed bridgework and/or removable partial dentures often provide acceptable results. However it is to the patient's advantage that implants be considered in a comparable light with conventional restorations.

Following through the premise set in chapter 4, that *the ideal restoration should not be compromised by the cause of tooth loss and should itself not compromise general dental health*, it is possible that conventional prostheses may themselves be contraindicated. Typically, in a young patient with unrestored abutment teeth, a conventional fixed bridge would be ill-advised.

In the case presented in this chapter, the patient suffered parasymphyseal mandibular fracture, loss of alveolus, and avulsion of four anterior teeth $\overline{3\ 2\ 1\ |\ 1}$ (43 42 41 31), with associated $\underline{\text{fracture}}$ of adjacent crowns on $\overline{5\ 4\ |\ 2\ 3}$ (45 44 32 33). There was a through and through horizontal split of the lip, associated with the direct trauma from hitting the steering wheel in a road traffic accident.

It was apparent that substantial bone loss and scarring were likely to

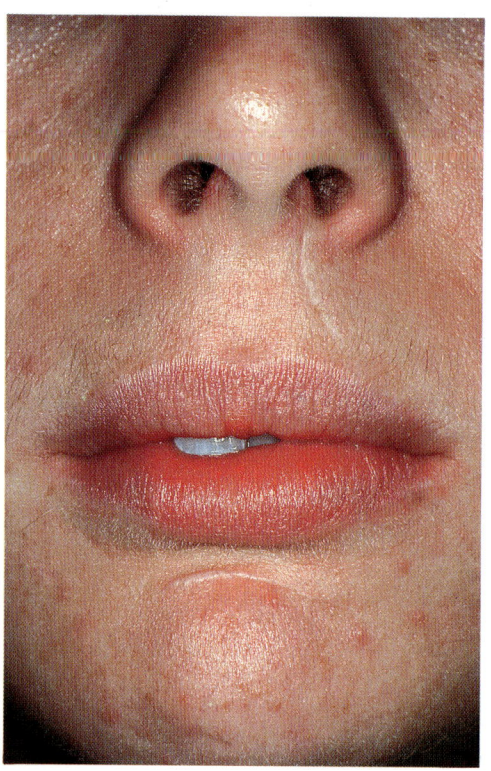

Fig 6-3 Loss of teeth and alveolus, in combination with intra- and extra-oral scarring, has resulted in loss of lip contour. The labio-mentalis groove has deepened, with subsequent trapping of the lower lip behind the upper central incisor.

compromise the construction of an aesthetic conventional fixed bridge, which the patient would have been unable to clean and may have inadequately restored lip support (Fig 6-3). Furthermore the patient presented with a heavy bite, which would easily destabilise a removable partial denture.

A decision was taken to restore the patient with a hybrid prosthesis supported by means of implants placed in the residual alveolus (Fig 6-4). A diagnostic wax set up clearly indicates the poor position of the implants in relation to the arch line (Fig 6-5), as dictated by the residual ridge morphology.

A cast substructure (Fig 6-6) was constructed on precision fit cylinders and screw retained to the implants, splinting them according to the principles set out by Lothigius et al.[1,2] Two Mini Conex (Cendres et Métaux SA Biel, Switzerland) attachments were cantilevered labially, the patrix parts being located within the Co/Cr framework of the partial overdenture (Fig 6-7).

When activated, the precision attachments provide the essential retention required for the prosthesis

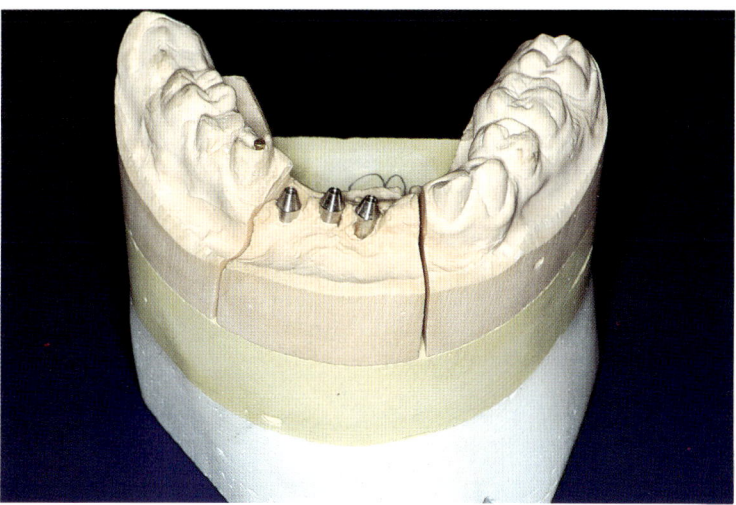

Fig 6-4 The master cast demonstrates the position of implants, placed in the residual alveolus after removal of bone plates used to reduce the fracture.

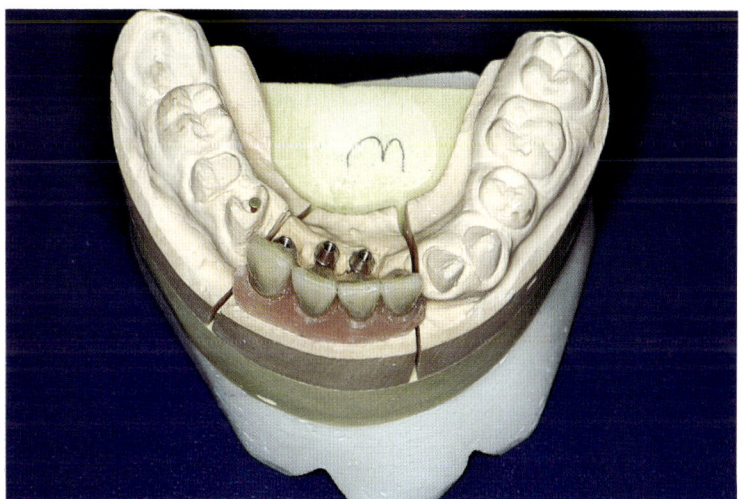

Fig 6-5 As a result of residual ridge morphology implants can be seen to be lingually placed in relation to the wax set-up, which represents the ideal position for dental and soft tissue rehabilitation. It was on this basis, that the decision was taken to fabricate a hybrid prosthesis.

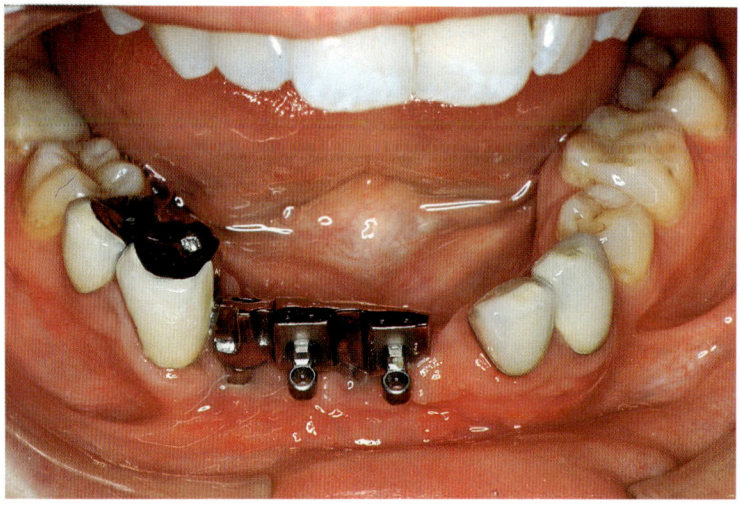

Fig 6-6 The milled substructure varies from the conventional design in shape and in the choice of precision attachment. In this case two Mini Conex attachments (Cendres et Métaux SA Biel, Switzerland) are labially cantilevered to provide retention under the incisal table.

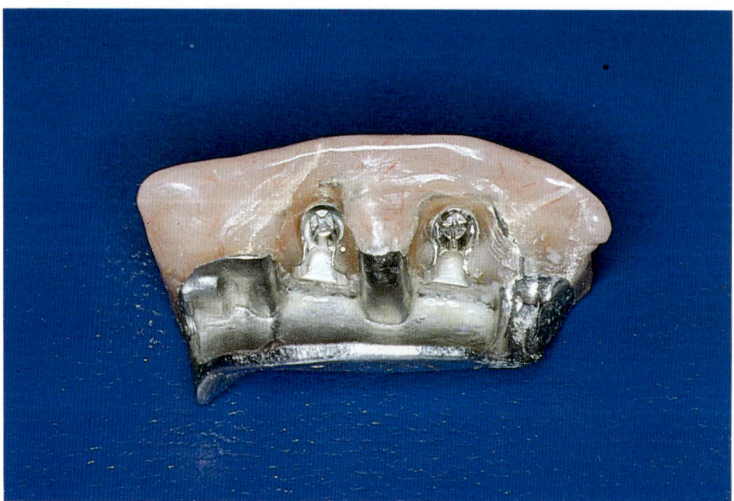

Fig 6-7 The fitting surface of this partial overdenture demonstrates the close fitting Cobalt/Chromium framework, which incorporates the male components of the Mini Conex attachments.

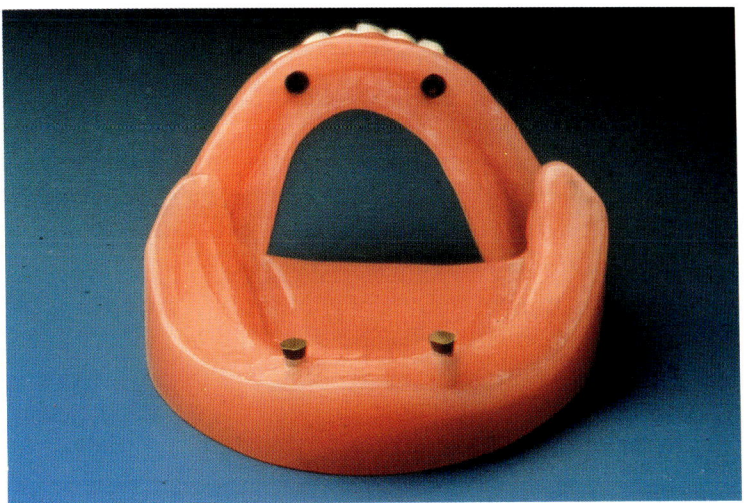

Fig 7-3 The model demonstrates the magnet attachment system for retention of an overdenture. The magnet keeper is screwed directly on to a 45° Uni-Abutment ™ and secured by bonding with a small drop of Ceka bond (Ceka NV, Antwerp, Belgium). The magnets are incorporated in to the fitting surface of the overdenture. Retentive power can not be altered.

reduction in implant success rates is noted in maxillary overdentures, though this is still comparable to data collated from maxillary fixed bridgework.

The biting forces created by an overdenture[12] are comparable, though in a lower range, than those created by fixed bridgework[13,14] and compare favourably to those created by a conventional denture.[15-17] However some concern arises as to the distribution of these forces to the underlying implants. An overdenture should derive some of its support from the underlying denture bearing area and as such horseshoe dentures are not recommended (as compared to the hybrid prosthesis). Studies have demonstrated that compressive and tensile forces on implants are reduced under an overdenture[18] whilst bending moments are higher as the denture causes flexion of the bar.[18] However, it is clear that the inclination and orientation of the implants are not critical with respect to complications arising as a result of function.[19]

Other attachment systems are also well documented, in particular, the ball and socket or retentive anchor attachment (Fig 7-2) which has been compared to overdentures supported by the bar and clip attachments.[8-10] These have been separately reported in short term prospective studies[20, 21] which have demonstrated high success rates in mandibular rehabilitation. Furthermore one study has shown a positive response at the periimplant and marginal bone level to the loading of these unsplinted fixtures,[21] which is comparable to other studies that have measured similar parameters in the bar and clip overdenture.[7, 9, 11]

However some reports[5, 8] and anecdotal evidence would appear to suggest that the ball and socket attachment should be confined to mandibular overdentures, where bicortical fixation is available to resist the high tensile forces imparted to the individual implants on withdrawing the denture.

A more recent free standing attachment, better suited to maxillary rehabilitation, is the magnet attachment (Fig 7-3). An overdenture can derive the necessary retention from magnet attachments, but not stability which must be provided through full coverage of the denture bearing area. The use of magnets to retain dentures is well documented[22-24] as is the subsequent problems of corrosion and loss of magnetism. However the recent publication of a 3-year prospective study on magnet retained overdentures demonstrates that such problems have been overcome by utilising a neodymium-iron-boron magnet, as compared to the historical cobalt samarium magnet.[25] Implant success rates with the magnets would seem comparable to both the ball and socket and the bar and clip attachment systems. However, data would suggest that free standing implants need to be at least 11 mm in length if they are to be able to withstand both the compressive and tensile forces of chewing and withdrawal of the denture.[25]

A distinct advantage of free standing attachment systems is that prophylaxis is facilitated and the patient is better able to maintain good periimplant health. Indeed, of all the possible restorations studied, the bar and clip retained overdenture has the highest recorded levels for periimplant complications, in particular mucosal hyperplasia.[5, 11, 26]

Treatment procedures

These are designed to reflect the simplicity of the overdenture modality, with clinical and technical requirements proving less demanding than for full fixed bridgework. Nonetheless, the clinician would be well advised to follow through a full clinical programme that includes articulation on a semi-adjustable articulator and try-in of dentures prior to insertion.

It is clear that a patient who presents with unsuccessful dentures, as in figure 7-4, may only require a degree of professional care to provide an optimised set of conventional dentures that offer a better fit and a more balanced occlusion. A great deal of information can be learnt from previous sets of dentures, such as hygiene ability and patient tolerance, which is often reflected by the number of sets the patient has in their shopping bag!!

It is important that an evaluation of the patient's requirements are well understood. If aesthetics alone are the source of disquiet, this may not necessarily be improved by implant support. A patient treatment planned for implants to solve such a presenting complaint may well prove dissatisfied with the result, even if chewing efficiency is markedly improved.

For bar splinted implants, impression techniques are the same as for fixed bridge reconstruction utilising direct impression copings, abutments and cylinders (see chapter 5). The laboratory technique only varies in that the bar is usually prefabricated rather than cast and as such it is soldered to the prefabricated cylinders (Fig 7 - 5). For the ball (Fig 7 - 6) and magnet (Fig 7 - 7) attachments, the Astra Tech system recommends the use of the 45° Uni-Abutment™ (Fig 3 - 9), which acts to reduce the vertical infringement of the implant/abutment complex on the bulk of the denture. This compares to the bar splinted technique in which the vertical height of a bar and clip may compromise the available interocclusal space and hence the strength and bulk of the overdenture. As such it may be necessary to provide additional strength by means of a thinner palatal or lingual Co/Cr veneer.

Impression techniques for the ball and magnet also vary, in that impressions are taken of the attachments themselves and not the abutments.

For the ball and socket a ball impression coping is placed over the ball attachment (Fig 7 - 8), which is screwed directly to the abutment and additionally secured by the use of a bonding agent, such as cyanoacrylate or Ceka Bond (Ceka NV, Antwerp, Belgium). Another alternative, is to use a one piece ball abutment, which screws directly into the fixture.

The copings remain within the impression on withdrawal. Ball abutment replicas can now be placed into the impression and incorporated into the master cast (Fig 7 - 9).

For the magnet attachment, techniques are further simplified, with an elastic or hydrocolloid impression being taken directly over the magnet keepers, which are secured to the abutments in a similar manner. On pouring up the master cast, stone replicas are apparent (Fig 7 - 10).

For the bar and ball attachment systems, the opposing components are activated and secured into place on the master cast (Fig 7 - 11). For the magnet system, magnets are secured to the stone replicas by means of cyanoacrylate (Fig 7 - 12).

It is necessary to block out all undercuts and use spacers where indicated by the manufacturers. A baseplate incorporating the attachments is waxed up and processed in clear acrylic.

This protocol will allow an assessment of the accuracy of fit of the precision attachments, by means of a baseplate try-in (Fig 7 - 13). At this appointment it is necessary to determine not only the accurate location

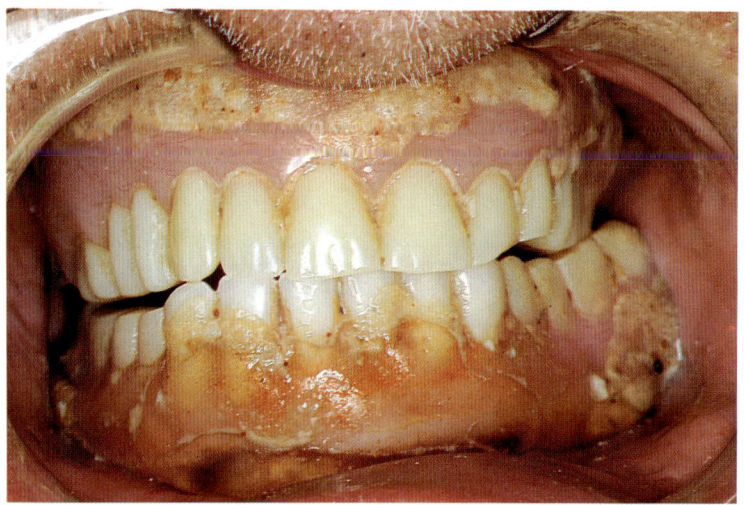

Fig 7-4 A patient who presents with dentures like those pictured above, may only need a degree of professional care to provide a new optimised set of conventional dentures. If problems still persist, it is then reasonable to treatment plan for implants.

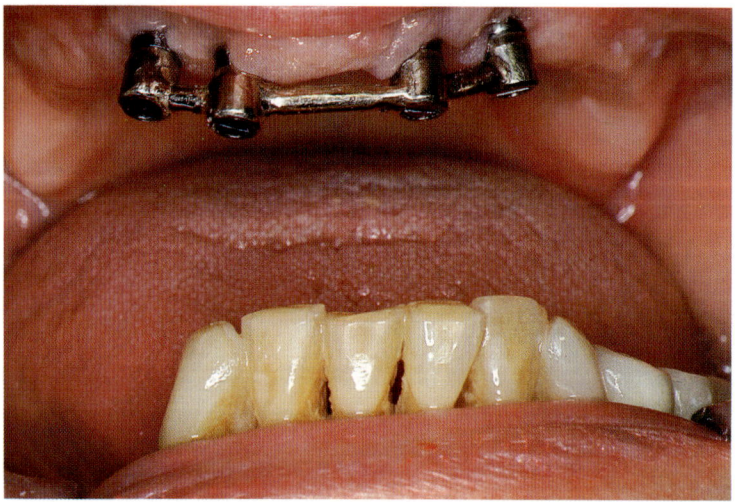

Fig 7-5 Prefabricated bars are usually available in 50 mm lengths. The bar is sectioned accordingly and soldered to the cylinders on the master model. A metalwork try-in will be necessary to ensure passive fit.

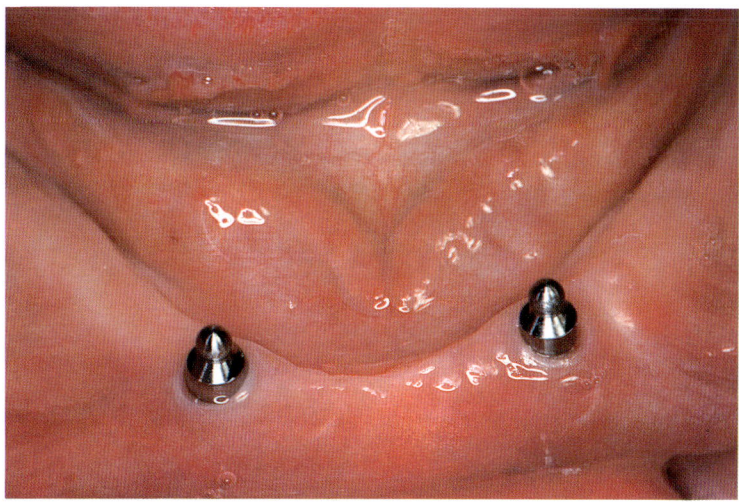

Fig 7-6 Ball attachments are ideally placed in the canine regions. Though two balls provide adequate retention, the placement of four balls prevents rocking of the denture, which can occur when the incisal table is anterior to the two balls.

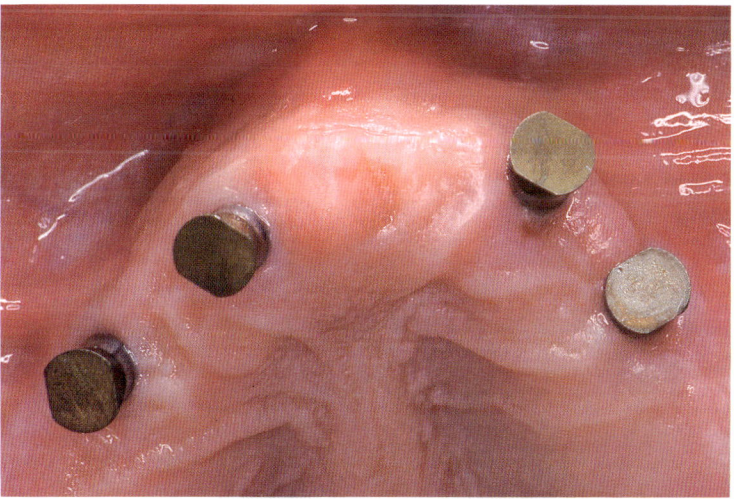

Fig 7-7 Position of implants for magnet attachments should be well spread with preferably two magnets in the premolar regions and two in the canine regions. In the case shown all four implants were placed in the premaxilla, which was only possible by means of a nasal floor lift procedure. The remaining maxilla was of "egg shell" thickness.

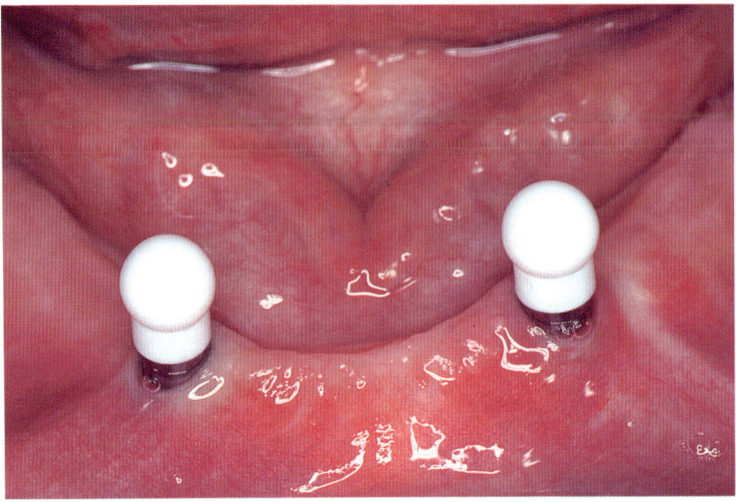

Fig 7-8a (above) and Fig 7-8b (below) show how the ball impression coping snaps over the ball attachment, but remains in the impression on withdrawal.

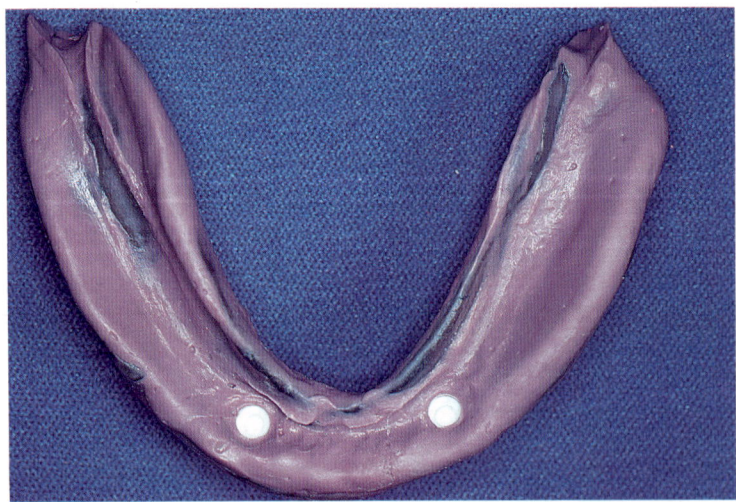

Fig 7-8b

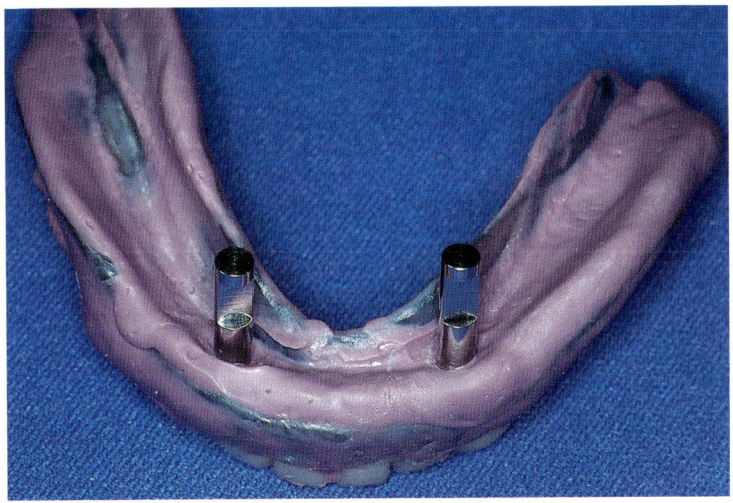

Fig 7-9 Laboratory ball analogues (ball replicas) are seated in to the ball impression copings, prior to casting. The master cast therefore incorporates balls that relate exactly to the clinical status.

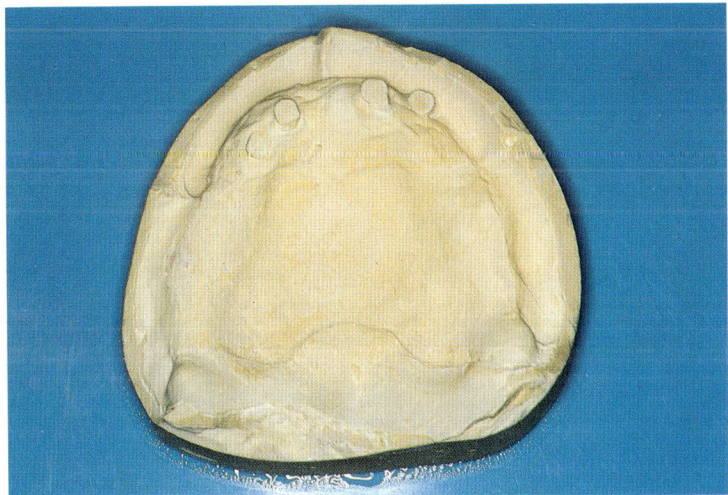

Fig 7-10 No analogues are required for the flat top magnet keeper. Instead a direct impression is cast, revealing stone replicas of the keepers. In an effort to increase the strength of the replicas, it is possible to pour cold cured acrylic into the impression of the keepers, prior to casting up.

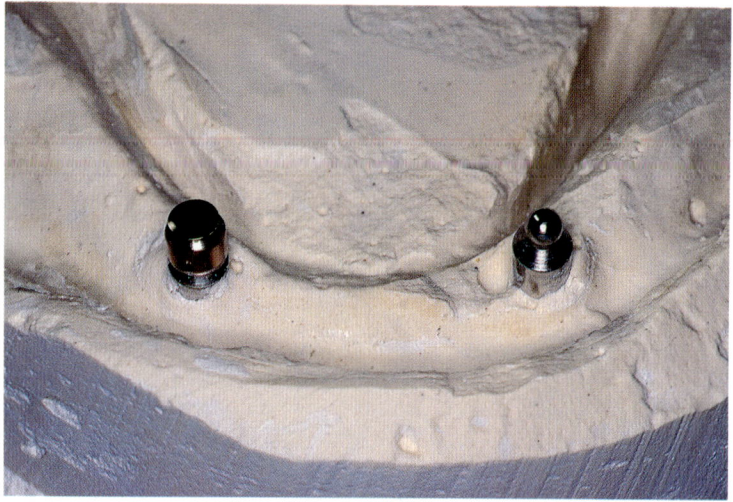

Fig 7-11 Clips for the bar and balls are activated on the bench top and located on the master cast. Spacers may be recommended by the manufacturers. All undercuts will need to be blocked out in plaster, prior to waxing up the baseplate.

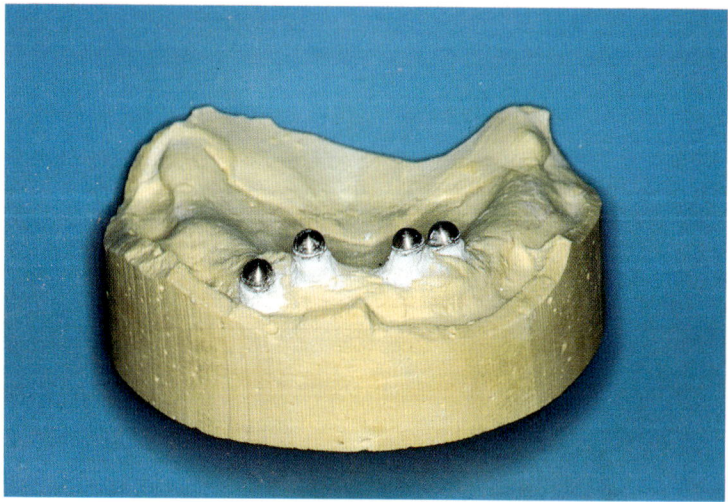

Fig 7-12 The magents are simply stuck to the stone or acrylic replicas using cyanoacrylate. The undercuts are blocked out in plaster prior to waxing up the baseplate.

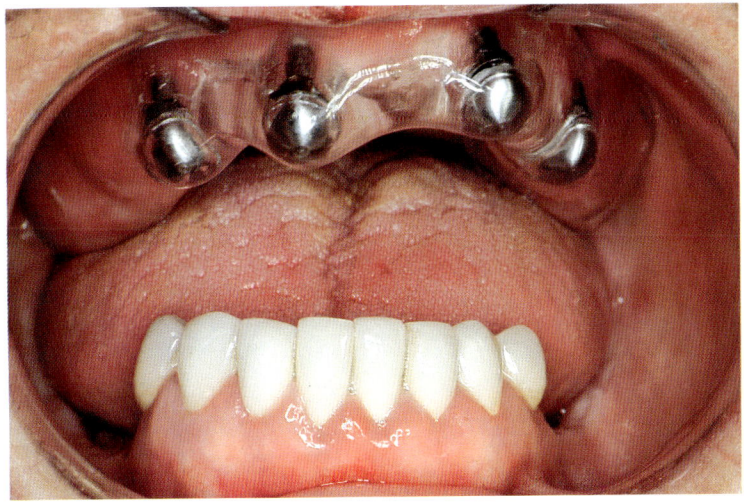

Fig 7-13 Baseplates should be cured in clear acrylic so that a baseplate try-in will reveal the accurate location of the attachments and the displacement of tissues in the denture bearing area.

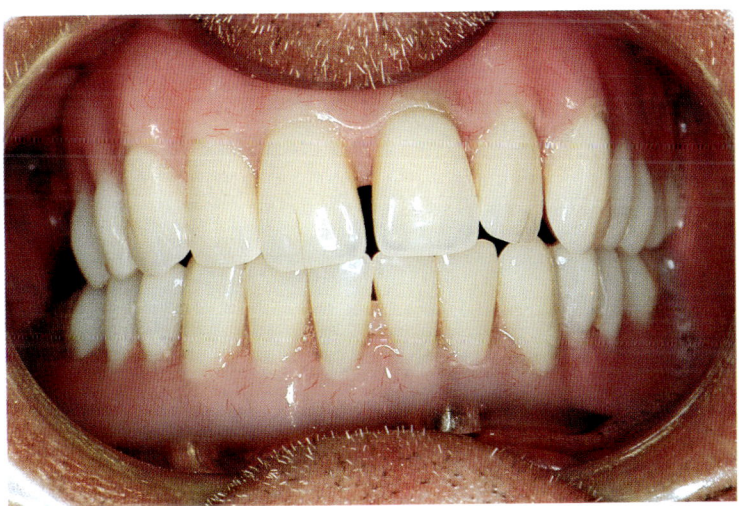

Fig 7-14 The incorporation of a midline diastema, slight imbrication or other imperfections will often serve to personalise the otherwise regimental set up so often characteristic of the standard denture. A balanced occlusion at the correct vertical dimension is of course paramount.

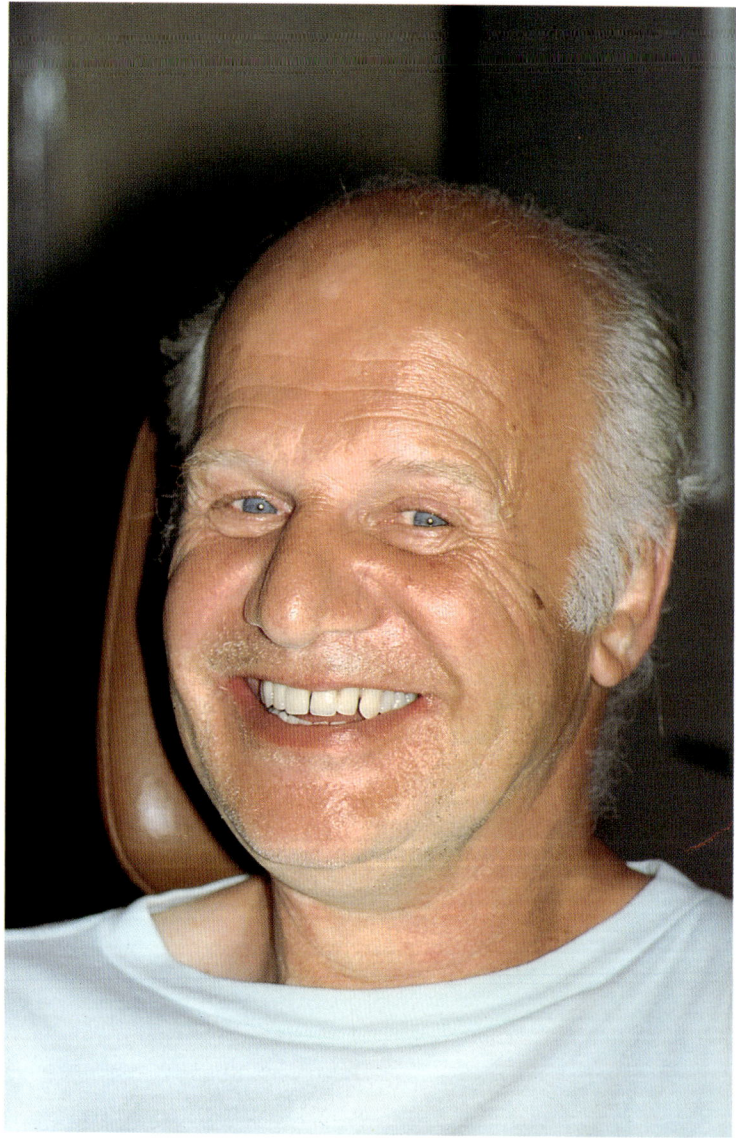

Fig 7-15 Aesthetics are defined not only by the textbook ideal, but by patient preference. The patient should be encouraged to take an active role in determining the final aesthetic result.

of the attachments but also the overall displacement of soft tissues in the denture bearing areas. The patient is afforded the first opportunity to appreciate the retentive powers of the future overdenture.

In addition to baseplate try-in, a metalwork try-in is also indicated for bar splinted overdentures in order to assess passive fit. Any evidence of poor location of one or more cylinders, or the presence of pressure on securing the bar to the abutments, will necessitate sectioning, indexing and resoldering of the bar. Subsequent repositioning of the clips in the baseplate may also be necessary.

It is now possible to add wax occlusal rims and proceed with bite registration as recommended in standard texts for the fabrication of conventional dentures.[27] It is of course essential to register the correct occlusal plane and vertical occlusal dimension, along with a recording of midline, high smile line and canine lines within the wax rim. Bite registration and wax try-in are facilitated by the presence of well retained baseplates.

The fabrication of aesthetic dentures that provide adequate soft tissue support is paramount and necessitates a wax try-in. To help achieve aesthetics that will serve to satisfy the patient, it is always useful to ask if any photographs are available showing the patient smiling with their natural teeth. Patients will often comment that they do not wish to reproduce the look of their natural teeth, however it can be equally as useful to know what the patient does not want by provision of the same photograph.

The incorporation of a midline diastema, slight imbrication or other imperfections will often serve to personalise the otherwise regimental set up so often characteristic of the standard denture (Fig 7-14). The inclusion of amalgam restorations, may also lend a more authentic character to the occlusal table.

The insertion appointment should allow for an assessment of all parameters recorded during previous visits as listed in Table 7-2.

The patient will need to be instructed on how to remove the prosthesis in a manner that does not differentially load the supporting implants with unfavourable tensile forces. The prosthesis should be withdrawn by applying thumb pressure either to the midline or with equal pressure either side of the midline. On first attempt patients will often be alarmed at the degree of retention and the perception of tensile forces on the implants. However, they soon become accustomed, preferring to remove the denture themselves on subsequent appointments, rather than allowing the clinician to remove them.

Recall Appointments

These appointments should be arranged for one week, one month and then six monthly. It will not be uncommon for the patient to complain of pressure sores after the first week. These should be highlight-

125

Table 7-2   Check List on Insertion of Overdentures

1   Check degree of clasp activation prior to insertion.

2   Ensure clasps or magnets accurately locate on the attachments on insertion.

3   Assess "fit" of the prosthesis over the denture bearing area, in particular denture extension and presence of pressure spots. (Adjust accordingly.)

4   Ensure that occlusion is well balanced and that the occlusal table is at the correct occlusal vertical dimension. Measure freeway space.

5   Seek the patient's assessment of aesthetics (Fig 7-15).

6   Check phonetics.

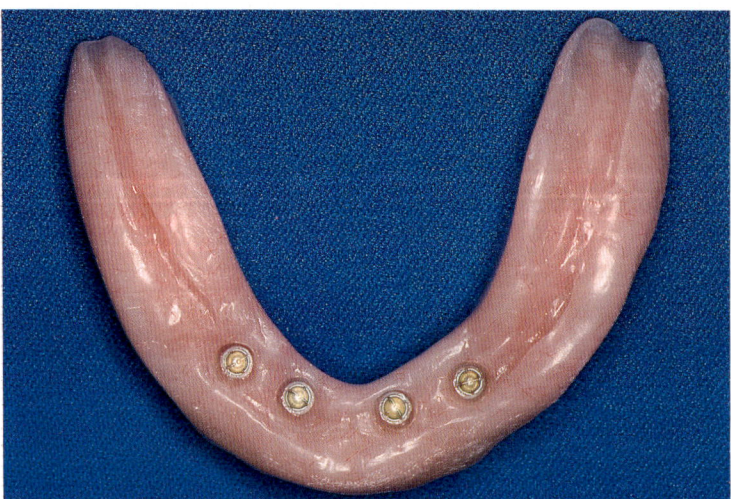

Fig 7-16 Ball clips are cross cut and can be reactivated or deactivated with special instruments, that crimp or splay the flanges.

porting overdentures in the mandible. A 2-year follow-up study. Clin Oral Impl Res 1993; 4: 83-89.

22 *Behrman, S.J.* The implantation of magnets in the jaw to aid retention. J Prosthet Dent 1960; 10: 807-841.

23 *Gorvey, S., Smuckler, H.* The full lower magnetic implant. J Dent Assoc S Afr 1961; 16: 365-368.

24 *Laird, W.R.E., Smith, G.A., Grant, A.A.* The use of magnetic forces in prosthetic dentistry. J Dent 1981; 9: 328-335.

25 *Walmsley, A.D., Brady, C.L., Smith, P.L., Frame, J.W.* Magnet retained overdentures using the Astra dental implant system. Br Dent J 1993; 174: 399-404.

26 *Jemt, T., Book, K., Lindén, B., Urde, G.* Failures and complications in 92 consecutively inserted overdentures supported by Brånemark implants in severely resorbed edentulous maxillae: A study from prosthetic treatment to first annual check-up. Int J Oral Maxillofac Implants 1992; 7: 162-167.

27 *Watt, D.M., MacGregor, A.R.* Designing complete dentures. Philadelphia: W.B. Saunders Company, 1976.

28 *Grogono, A.L., Lancaster, D.M., Finger, I.M.* Dental implants: A survey of patient's attitudes. J Prosthet Dent 1989; 62: 573-576.

29 *Kiyak, H.A., Beach, B.H., Worthington, P., Taylor, T., Bolender, C., Evans, J.* The psychological impact of osseointegrated dental implants. Int J Oral Maxillofac Implants 1990; 5: 61-69.

30 *Blomberg, S., Lindquist, L.W.* Psychological reactions to edentulousness and treatment with jawbone-anchored bridges. Acta Psychiatr Scand 1983; 68: 251-262.

8 Post Insertion Maintenance

Prior to embarking on treatment with implants, it is important that the patient is fully aware of the commitment that is required, not only during treatment, but in the long term maintenance of the prosthesis.

It is the role of the practitioner to emphasise the need for six monthly or annual visits. An assessment of the continuing viability of both the prosthesis and the implants, from both a clinical and radiographic perspective, should be carried out.

There is some disagreement amongst clinicians as to whether or not there is a need to remove fixed prostheses on an annual basis, in order to assess the presence or absence of mobility of the supporting implants. Though there is some desire to do this, the removal of the prosthesis will often result in patient disapproval, which will occasionally prove well founded when, subsequent to prosthesis removal, problems occur in reseating the bridgework in exactly the same way.

Experience shows that in the absence of periimplant radiolucency and other clinical signs, mobility is unlikely. On balance it may prove wiser to remove the prosthesis only when clinical conditions dictate and not on an elective basis.

A paralleling technique is advisable when taking intra-oral radiographs, so that the threads appear in focus (Fig 8-1) since only then is it possible to determine a true periimplant radiolucency (Fig 8-2). Focusing on the marginal bone may demonstrate signs of crestal bone loss. Given that a radiograph is merely a picture in time, it is necessary to compare two or more radiographs over the first one to two years (Figs 8-3, 8-4a and 8-4b).

It is not unusual to have to re tighten bridge screws which may work loose during early functional loading of the bridge. This would seem to arise more commonly with those implants that utilise a butt joint interface.

Bridge screws that continue to present loose on subsequent recall appointments should arouse concern for the accuracy of fit of the bridgework, or possibly for overloading of the prosthesis. However, the advantage of the bridge screws being the weakest link in the chain is that not only do they act to protect the

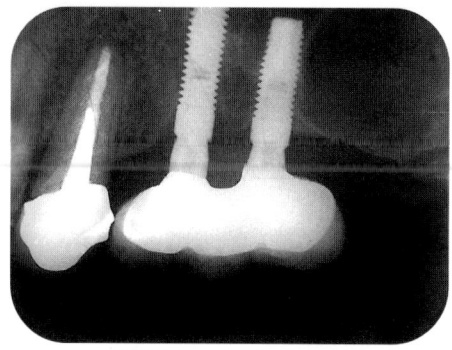

Fig 8-1 The use of a reproducible paralleling technique will ensure that the threads of the fixture are in focus. This is essential for accurate assessment of osseointegration or periimplant radiolucency.

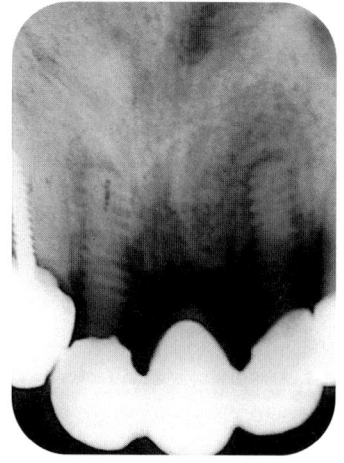

Fig 8-2 Periimplant radiolucency, seen here around two single crystal sapphire implants is characterised by a dark line that can be traced around the apex of the fixture, with no evidence of bone between the threads. This is a cardinal sign of implant failure.

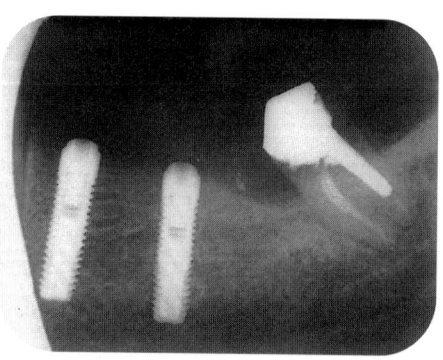

Fig 8-3 Radiographs should be taken prior to implant exposure to act as a baseline by which to compare future radiographs.

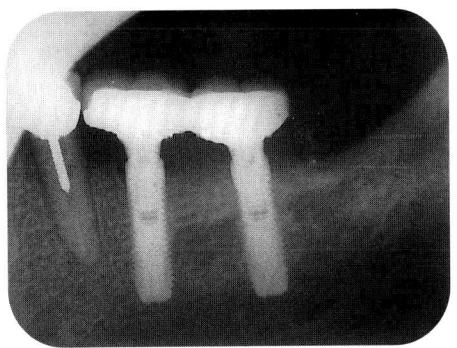

Fig 8-4a This radiograph was taken approximately 8 months post insertion. Note the molar seen in figure 8-3 was extracted and no socket remnant is now visible. When comparing the two radiographs it is clear that there has been a small cratering around the mesial aspect of the mesial implant. Future radiographic monitoring will determine if this is "physiological" or "pathological".

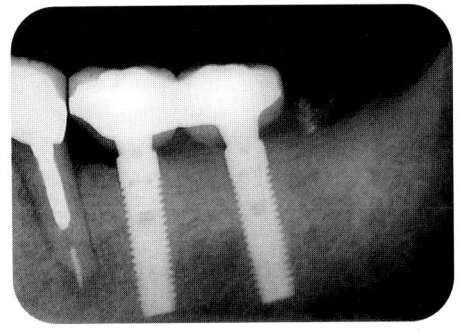

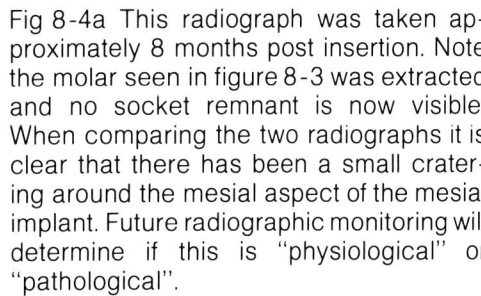

Fig 8-4b This radiograph was taken 2 years post insertion. Careful study of the bone around the mesial implant clearly demonstrates that the vertical bone loss seen in figure 8-4a has been stabilised and the crater filled with bone that is now visibly horizontal. This is indicative of a favourable load distribution by the prosthesis.

underlying implant/abutment complex but, being occlusally placed they are more easily accessed.

Considering that the majority of prospective studies cited in this text report a 100% prosthetic success (as compared to implant success), it is clear that having passed the first annual recall, the number of failures take a dramatic drop, statistically. Expected failures fall even further after the three and five year recall with only occasional case reports of long standing prostheses being compromised by implant failures.

The role of the hygienist may prove more critical during maintenance visits, bearing in mind that many implant patients lost their own teeth initially through poor dental health motivation. It is perhaps surprising that, with all the physical and financial investment involved in implant therapy, some patients still persist in ignoring oral hygiene instruction.

The presence of a plaque induced periimplant inflammatory response has been well documented[1, 2] and shown to be potentially destructive.[2] Studies show that it is not acceptable to clean the surface of abutments with standard metal scalers or ultrasonic instruments since these result in visual damage of the softer

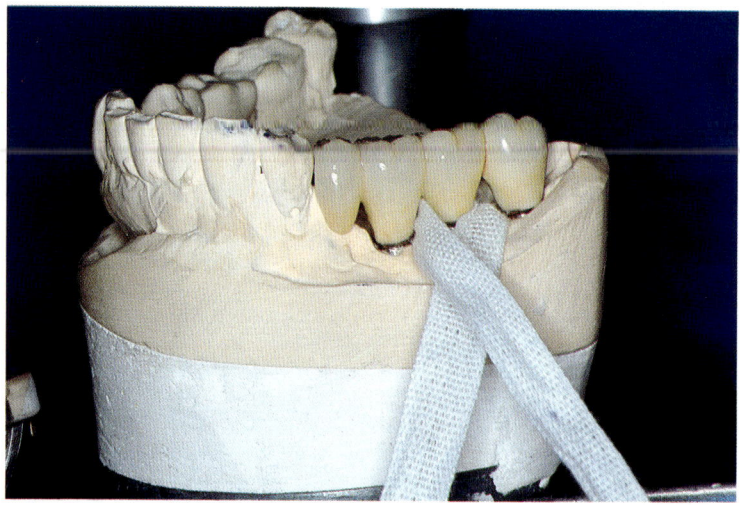

Fig 8-5 G-Floss II™ (3i™, Implant Innovations™, Palm Beach, Florida) is a type of ribbon floss which is very useful for cleaning around the necks of implants and in the interproximal spaces.

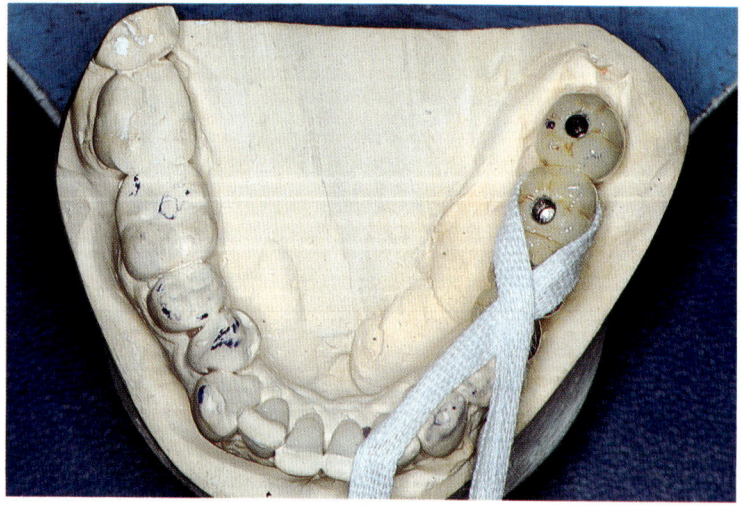

Fig 8-6 G-Floss II™ (3i™, Implant Innovations™, Palm Beach, Florida) is also useful for cleaning around the undersurface and the lingual surface of the bridgework.

titanium surface.[3-5] Instead the use of plastic scalers[6-9] or gold alloy scalers (Implarette Scaler™, 3i™ Implant Innovations™, Palm Beach, Florida) have been used to remove gross debris from abutment surfaces, without scratching or pitting the titanium.

In an effort to further remove debris, whilst leaving a polished surface, investigators have studied the effects of abrasive pastes applied by rubber cup;[6, 7] air-powder abrasive systems;[5, 6, 10] and flour of pumice, applied by rubber cup.[5, 10] The flour of pumice applied intermittently, with light pressure, would seem to provide the best results with obliteration of the machine milling marks, leaving a smooth swirl pattern.[10] This prophylactic technique is also easily accessible to the general practice hygienist.

The most important job for both dentist and hygienist is to convey a sense of encouragement to the patient. The role of the patient in his or her long term maintenance programme is of paramount importance. The use of soft tooth brushes and interdental brushes is to be recommended, though without the use of toothpaste, which can prove too abrasive for the softer titanium.

The use of floss and super floss are of limited value around the larger gaps, and the bulky fixed bridge prosthesis. However, the introduction of G-Floss™ (3i™, Implant Innovations™, Palm Beach, Florida) allows more effective cleaning in those awkward nooks and crannies (Figs 8-5 and 8-6).

Above all the patient should be encouraged to possess a high level of awareness for the feel and function of the prosthesis. It should be abundantly clear that at the first sign of trouble or even concern, the patient should present for a check-up. The result of procrastination will often be that a minor complication is now more costly, in all respects!!

Perhaps the most significant advantage of regular maintenance appointments is the constant reminder of both the predictability of implants and the total improvement in quality of life that such restorations can provide.

References

1   Berglundh, T., Lindhe, J., Marinello, C., Ericsson, I., Liljenberg, B. Soft tissue reaction to de novo plaque formation on implants and teeth. An experimental study in the dog. Clin Oral Impl Res 1992; 3: 1-8.

2   Ericsson, I., Berglundh, T., Marinello, C., Liljenberg, B., Lindhe, J. Long-standing plaque and gingivitis at implants and teeth in the dog. Clin Oral Impl Res 1992; 3: 99-103.

3   Thomson-Neal, D., Evans, G.H., Meffert, R.M. Effects of various prophylactic treatments on titanium, sapphire, and hydroxyapatite-coated implants: An SEM study. Int J Periodont Rest Dent 1989; 9: 301-311.

4   Fox, S.C., Moriarty, J.D., Kusy, R.P. The effects of scaling a titanium implant surface with metal and plastic instruments: An in vitro study. J Periodontol 1990; 61: 485-490.

5   Rapley, J.W., Swan, R.H., Hallmon, W.W., Mills, M.P. The surface characteristics produced by various oral hygiene instruments and materials on titanium implant abutments. Int J Oral Maxillofac Implants 1990; 5: 47-52.

6   Stefani, L. The care and maintenance of the dental implant patient. J Dent Hygiene 1988; 62: 477.

7   Orton, G.S., Steele, D.L., Wolinsky, L.E. The dental professional's role in monitoring and maintenance of tissue-integrated prostheses. Int J Oral Maxillofac Implants 1989; 4: 305-310.

8   Brough, K., Johnson, R., Carr, P., Daffron, P. The dental hygienist's role in the maintenance of osseointegrated dental implants. J Dent Hygiene 1988; 62: 448.

9   Balshi, T.J. Hygiene maintenance procedures for patients treated with the tissue integrated prosthesis (osseointegration). Quintessence Int 1986; 17: 95-102.

10 McCollum, J., O'Neal, R.B., Brennan, W.A., van Dyke, T.E., Horner, J.A. The effect of titanium implant abutment surface irregularities on plaque accumulation in vivo. J Periodontol 1992; 63: 802-805.

Retentive anchor Another term for the ball attachment system for overdentures.

Ridge mapping The measurement of bony ridge thickness in the surgical field.

Root form Description of shape. Pertaining to the implant.

Screw retrievable A fixed bridge which is made removable by means of unscrewing bridge screws made accessible through the occlusal surfaces of the bridgework.

Self tapping Refers to the implant which does not require the bone to be tapped prior to insertion.

Submerged Refers to the implant variety which is left beneath the mucoperiosteum during the healing phase.

Surgical stent See surgical template.

Surgical template Acrylic copy of diagnostic wax up, used during surgery to position the implants correctly.

Tapping Effected by a bone tap; this is the cutting of a thread directly into the bone prior to implant insertion.

Thermal trauma Referring to the osseonecrosis that can be caused by drilling heats that exceed 47°C for 1 minute.

TiOblast™ A technique by which an implant surface is roughened by blasting with TiO_2 particles (Astra Tech AB, Mölndal, Sweden).

Titanium Plasma Spray (TPS) A coating approximately $30\mu m$ thick, on the surface of an implant, which creates a rough layer thought to help increase bone apposition.

TME Transmucosal element. See abutment.

Torque controller Instrument used to unite various components by applying a prescribed torque to create a pretension in the abutment and bridge screws.

Torque forces Rotational forces which when applied to a fixture may have the effect of fracturing the bone/implant interface. The use of torque forces have been applied to measuring the resistance of an implant to being unscrewed from bone (40-150 Ncm).

Transfer template Acrylic jig used to transfer unsplinted copings from the master cast to the mouth in their correct orientation.

Transitional prosthesis An all acrylic temporary prosthesis used to progressively load implants prior to insertion of a permanent restoration.

Transmucosal Refers to the implant variety which is left exposed in the mouth, with the implant neck penetrating the mucosa.

Transmucosal collar The body of a two part abutment. It is secured to the fixture by means of an abutment screw.

Trephine drills These are burs used for cutting troughs, with a central core, in bone to receive a hollow basket type implant. Trephines are also used for the complete removal of implants when they need to be cut out of bone.

True Bone Height As compared to bone height measured on a radiograph, which may be distorted.

Twist drill These are burs used for cutting cylindrical preparations in bone to receive a solid screw or press fit implant.

Two stage procedure Refers to submerged implants, where a second surgical procedure is required to expose the implants.

Uni-abutment™ Refers to the one piece final abutment specific to the Astra Tech implant system.

Index